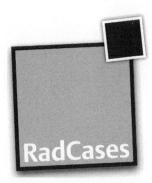

Musculoskeletal Radiology

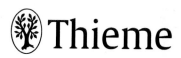

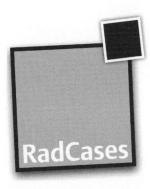

Musculoskeletal Radiology

Edited by

Glenn M. Garcia, MD
Assistant Professor
Section of Musculoskeletal Imaging
Department of Radiology
The University of Texas Health Science Center at San Antonio
San Antonio, Texas

Series Editors

Jonathan Lorenz, MD
Associate Professor of Radiology
Department of Radiology
The University of Chicago
Chicago, Illinois

Hector Ferral, MD
Professor of Radiology
Section Chief, Interventional Radiology
Rush University Medical Center, Chicago
Chicago, Illinois

Thieme
New York • Stuttgart

Thieme Medical Publishers, Inc.
333 Seventh Ave.
New York, NY 10001

Executive Editor: Timothy Hiscock
Editorial Director: Michael Wachinger
Editorial Assistant: Adriana di Giorgio
International Production Director: Andreas Schabert
Production Editor: Katy Whipple, Maryland Composition
Vice President, International Marketing and Sales: Cornelia Schulze
Chief Financial Officer: James W. Mitos
President: Brian D. Scanlan
Compositor: MPS Content Services
Printer: Maple-Vail Book Manufacturing Group

Library of Congress Cataloging-in-Publication Data

Musculoskeletal radiology / edited by G. Garcia.
    p. ; cm. — (RadCases)
  Includes bibliographical references and index.
  ISBN 978-1-60406-179-6
  1. Musculoskeletal system — Radiography — Case studies. I. Garcia, G. (Glenn) II. Series: RadCases.

  [DNLM: 1. Musculoskeletal Diseases--radiography — Case Reports. 2. Diagnosis, Differential — Case Reports. 3. Musculoskeletal System — radiography — Case Reports. WE 141 M985856 2010]
  RC925.7.M878 2010
  616.7'07548 — dc22
                    2009038135

Important note: Medical knowledge is ever-changing. As new research and clinical experience broaden our knowledge, changes in treatment and drug therapy may be required. The authors and editors of the material herein have consulted sources believed to be reliable in their efforts to provide information that is complete and in accord with the standards accepted at the time of publication. However, in view of the possibility of human error by the authors, editors, or publisher of the work herein or changes in medical knowledge, neither the authors, editors, nor publisher, nor any other party who has been involved in the preparation of this work, warrants that the information contained herein is in every respect accurate or complete, and they are not responsible for any errors or omissions or for the results obtained from use of such information. Readers are encouraged to confirm the information contained herein with other sources. For example, readers are advised to check the product information sheet included in the package of each drug they plan to administer to be certain that the information contained in this publication is accurate and that changes have not been made in the recommended dose or in the contraindications for administration. This recommendation is of particular importance in connection with new or infrequently used drugs.

Some of the product names, patents, and registered designs referred to in this book are in fact registered trademarks or proprietary names even though specific reference to this fact is not always made in the text. Therefore, the appearance of a name without designation as proprietary is not to be construed as a representation by the publisher that it is in the public domain.

Printed in the United States

978-1-60406-179-6

To my daughter Claire, who melts my heart. To my wife Kelley, for her endless support.
—Glenn Garcia

Series Preface

The ability to assimilate detailed information across the entire spectrum of radiology is the Holy Grail sought by those preparing for their trip to Louisville. As enthusiastic partners in the Thieme RadCases series who formerly took the examination, we understand the exhaustion and frustration shared by residents and the families of residents engaged in this quest. It has been our observation that despite ongoing efforts to improve Web-based interactive databases, residents still find themselves searching for material they can review while preparing for the radiology board examinations and remain frustrated by the fact that only a few printed guidebooks are available, which are limited in both format and image quality. Perhaps their greatest source of frustration is the inability to easily locate groups of cases across all subspecialties of radiology that are organized and tailored for their immediate study needs. Imagine being able to immediately access groups of high-quality cases to arrange study sessions, quickly extract and master information, and prepare for theme-based radiology conferences. Our goal in creating the RadCases series was to combine the popularity and portability of printed books with the adaptability, exceptional quality, and interactive features of an electronic case-based format.

The intent of the printed book is to encourage repeated priming in the use of critical information by providing a portable group of exceptional core cases that the resident can master. The best way to determine the format for these cases was to ask residents from around the country to weigh in. Overwhelmingly, the residents said that they would prefer a concise, point-by-point presentation of the Essential Facts of each case in an easy-to-read, bulleted format. Differentials are limited to a maximum of three, and the first is always the actual diagnosis. This approach is easy on exhausted eyes and provides a quick review of Pearls and Pitfalls as information is absorbed during repeated study sessions. We worked hard to choose cases that could be presented well in this format, recognizing the limitations inherent in reproducing high-quality images in print. Unlike the authors of other case-based radiology review books, we removed the guesswork by providing clear annotations and descriptions for all images. In our opinion, there is nothing worse than being unable to locate a subtle finding on a poorly reproduced image even after one knows the final diagnosis.

The electronic cases expand on the printed book and provide a comprehensive review of the entire subspecialty. Thousands of cases are strategically designed to increase the resident's knowledge by providing exposure to additional case examples-from basic to advanced-and by exploring "Aunt Minnie's," unusual diagnoses, and variability within a single diagnosis. The search engine gives the resident a fighting chance to find the Holy Grail by creating individualized, daily study lists that are not limited by factors such as radiology subsection. For example, tailor today's study list to cases involving tuberculosis and include cases in every subspecialty and every system of the body. Or study only thoracic cases, including those with links to cardiology, nuclear medicine, and pediatrics. Or study only musculoskeletal cases. The choice is yours.

As enthusiastic partners in this project, we started small and, with the encouragement, talent, and guidance of Tim Hiscock at Thieme, we have continued to raise the bar in our effort to assist residents in tackling the daunting task of assimilating massive amounts of information. We are passionate about continuing this journey, planning to expand the cases in our electronic series, adapt cases based on direct feedback from residents, and increase the features intended for board review and self-assessment. As the National Board of Medical Examiners converts the American Board of Radiology examination from an oral to an electronic format, our series will be the one best suited to meet the needs of the next generation of overworked and exhausted residents in radiology.

Jonathan Lorenz, MD
Hector Ferral, MD
Chicago, IL

Preface

The purpose of this book is to provide concise information regarding musculoskeletal imaging. Multimodality imaging of a variety of tumors, inflammatory conditions, metabolic disorders, traumatic injuries, infections, and congenital disorders are presented in a case-based format. The reader will be challenged with radiographs, magnetic resonance imaging, bone scan, and computed tomography. Every effort has been made to provide realistic clinical presentations, salient imaging findings, and reasonable differential diagnoses. Each case contains a brief summary of important and up-to-date clinical and radiologic facts. If the reader wishes to expand his or her knowledge, further readings for each case are included. It is the author's intent to provide the radiologist-in-training and/or the seasoned radiologist with a comprehensive, yet approachable, fund of knowledge in musculoskeletal imaging.

—*Glenn Garcia, MD*

Case 1

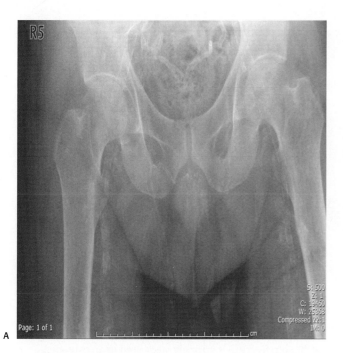

A

Clinical Presentation

An elderly woman who has experienced a fall is unable to bear weight on her right hip.

Further Work-up

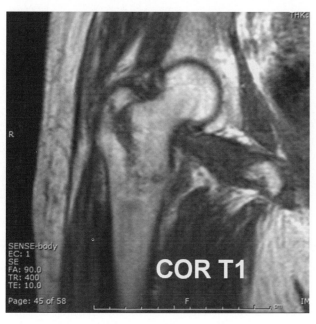

B

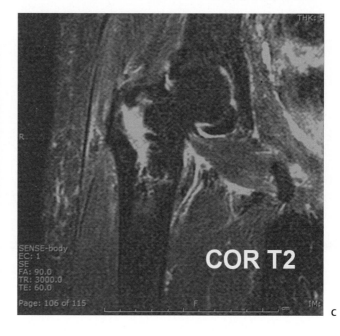

C

■ Imaging Findings

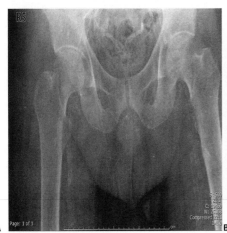 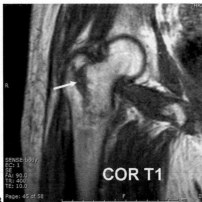 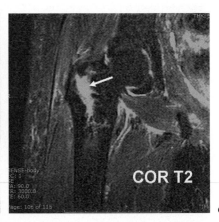

A   B   C

(A) Radiographic imaging of the hips shows heavily calcified arteries and osteopenia. No acute bony abnormality is seen. **(B,C)** Coronal magnetic resonance imaging (MRI) demonstrates an irregular focus of abnormally low signal intensity on the T1-weighted image and abnormally high signal intensity on the T2-weighted image (*arrows*) incompletely extending across the intertrochanteric region.

■ Differential Diagnosis

- **Nondisplaced incomplete intertrochanteric fracture:** Given the patient's presentation and the orientation and location of the derangement in the MRI signal, this diagnosis is most likely.
- *Insufficiency fracture:* The patient's history of a fall and the intertrochanteric location are not characteristic of this entity; insufficiency fractures favor the femoral neck.
- *Metastasis:* The lack of lobular masslike morphology is not typical of metastasis.

■ Essential Facts

- Nondisplaced, incomplete intertrochanteric and femoral neck hip fractures following a fall from a standing position are not uncommon in elderly female patients with osteopenia.
- The outcome of these fractures tends to be better if the fragments are not displaced.
- For this reason alone, MRI is necessary if such fractures are strongly suspected clinically in the setting of normal radiographic findings.

✔ Pearls & ✘ Pitfalls

- ✔ If a hip fracture is strongly suspected in an osteopenic patient with normal findings on plain radiographic films, limited coronal T1- and T2-weighted MRI is efficacious and can exclude a fracture. Characteristic findings of a fracture on MRI include irregular low T1-weighted and bright T2-weighted signal intensity.
- ✘ Occasionally, T2-weighted sequences may not adequately characterize the fracture secondary to surrounding edema/contusion.

Case 2

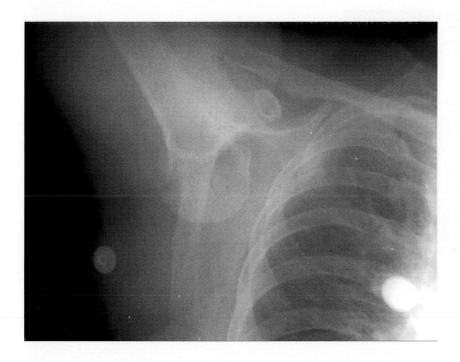

■ Clinical Presentation

The patient has sustained an injury while horseback riding.

■ Imaging Findings

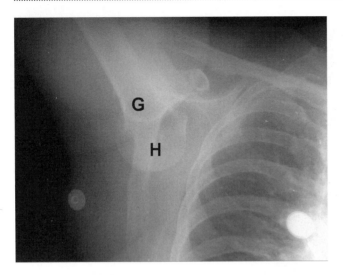

Frontal shoulder radiograph reveals inferior dislocation of the humerus (*H*) relative to the glenoid (*G*) with the arm hyperabducted.

■ Differential Diagnosis

- ***Luxatio erecta:*** This is represented by inferior dislocation of the shoulder, with the superior surface of the humeral head pointing inferiorly and not in contact with the glenoid fossa.
- *Anterior subcoracoid dislocation:* This is the most common anterior dislocation, in which the humeral head sits inferior to the coracoid process.
- *Subglenoid dislocation:* This is the second most common anterior dislocation, in which the superior surface of the humeral head is positioned inferior and slightly anterior to the glenoid fossa with the shoulder/arm adducted.

■ Essential Facts

- Luxatio erecta is a rare injury sustained when an axial load across an extended arm results from a direct force above the head.
- As a consequence, the arm is fixed over the head. Inferior capsular damage and neurovascular injuries can occur.
- Fractures of the coracoid process, acromion, inferior glenoid fossa, and humeral head have been described.

✔ Pearls & ✘ Pitfalls

- ✔ Patients with this injury exhibit a unique clinical presentation. The forearm is pronated and resting on the head. The humeral shaft is parallel to the scapular spine on the frontal radiograph.
- ✘ The injury can be misclassified as subglenoid anterior dislocation.

Case 3

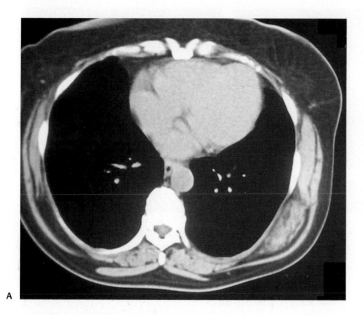

A

■ Clinical Presentation

....

The patient is a 65-year-old woman with a long history of a left-sided back mass.

Further Work-up

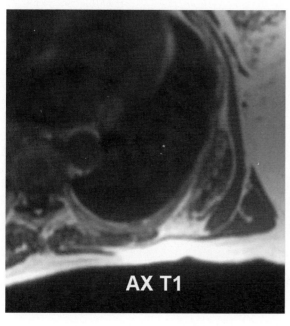

B

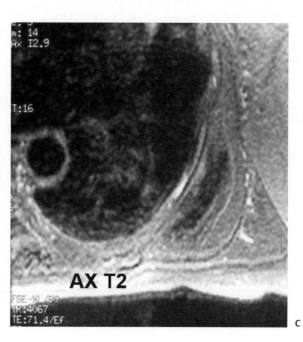

C

■ Imaging Findings

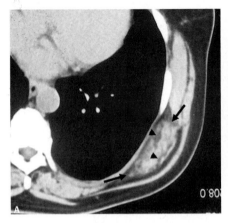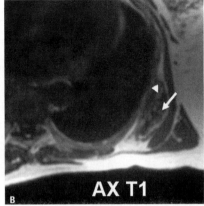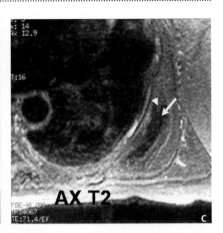

(A) A non–contrast-enhanced computed tomographic scan of the chest demonstrates a mass in the left posterior chest wall with muscle density (*long arrows*) and interstices of fat density (*arrowheads*). **(B,C)** Axial mag- netic resonance (MR) images through the mass show the lesion to contain predominantly areas of low signal intensity (*long arrows*) with correspond- ing areas of fat signal (*arrowheads*).

■ Differential Diagnosis

- **Elastofibroma:** The patient's age, location in the infra- scapular chest wall, and low-signal MR characteristics are diagnostic for this lesion.
- *Neurofibroma:* The MR signal characteristic of a target sign and the fusiform morphology are lacking in this case.
- *Lipoma:* Although there are areas of fat in this lesion, the location and signal characteristics are more typical of elas- tofibroma.

■ Essential Facts

- Elastofibroma is a degenerative, reactive, fibrous pseudo- tumor with abundant deposits of collagen, responsible for the MR characteristics. This lesion results from mechanical irritation and is usually seen in patients 55 years of age or older, who present with stiffness and pain.

✔ Pearls & ✘ Pitfalls

- ✔ Elastofibroma is commonly seen in the connective tissue between the posterior chest wall and inferomedial bor- der of the scapula, manifesting as a slowly growing mass. In 25% of cases, the lesions are bilateral.
- ✘ Although this is a benign process, the lesion may demon- strate uptake on positron emission tomography.

Case 4

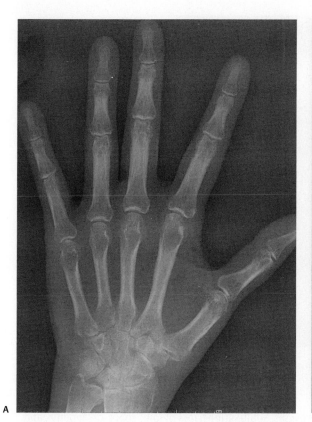
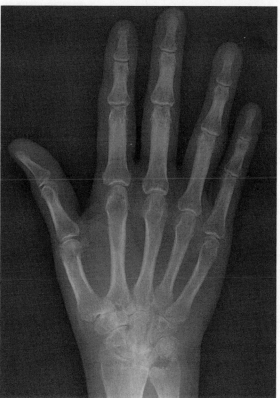

A   B

■ Clinical Presentation

The patient is a 50-year-old woman with polyarthralgias.

■ Imaging Findings

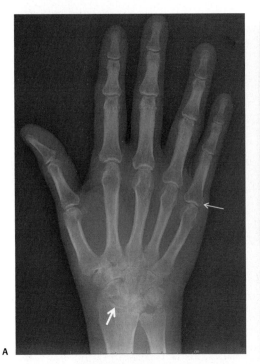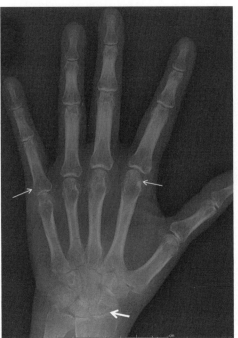

(A,B) Frontal radiographs of the hands show bilateral periarticular osteopenia (*thin arrows*) with loss of joint space across the wrist (*thick arrows*) joints and absence of osteophytes.

■ Differential Diagnosis

- *Rheumatoid arthritis (RA):* The female gender, symmetric distribution with periarticular osteopenia, and loss of wrist joint space are characteristic of RA.
- *Osteoarthritis:* Symmetric periarticular osteopenia and a diffuse loss of wrist joint space without osteophytes are not consistent with osteoarthritis.
- *Psoriatic arthritis:* The symmetry and distribution of findings with the absence of periostitis are not representative of psoriatic arthritis.

■ Essential Facts

- RA is a chronic, systemic polyarticular disease that predominantly involves synovial tissue and joints in a symmetric fashion.
- Circulating rheumatoid factor interacts with synovial membranes, eliciting inflammatory processes that are responsible for the arthropathic changes of periarticular erosions, subluxations, loss of joint space, osteopenia, and soft-tissue swelling.
- RA affects 0.5 to 1.0% of the global population, with women affected more frequently than men.
- Patients are typically 30 to 60 years of age.
- Symmetric involvement of the hands and wrists is common.
- Pancompartmental loss of wrist joint space is related to synovitis and may be seen in the absence of digit involvement.
- Ulnar styloid erosions and metacarpophalangeal (MCP) and proximal interphalangeal joint erosions with loss of joint space are typical.

✔ Pearls & ✘ Pitfalls

- ✔ The second and third MCP joints and the third proximal interphalangeal joint may be the first to exhibit findings of RA.
- ✘ Gout and lupus arthropathy may appear similar to RA in the hand and wrist.

Case 5

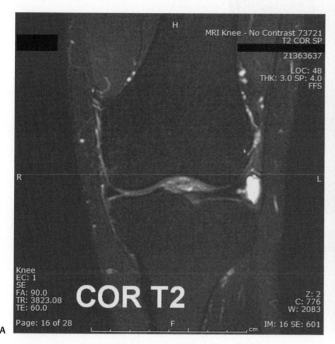
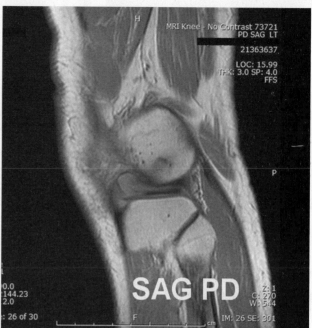

■ Clinical Presentation

The patient is a 26-year-old man with a palpable mass.

■ Imaging Findings

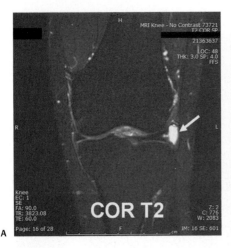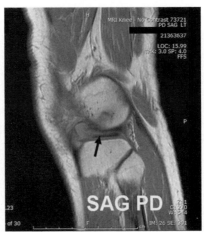

(A,B) Magnetic resonance (MR) images show a cystic lesion (*white arrow*) abutting the anterior horn of the lateral meniscus. The lesion is contiguous with a meniscal tear that extends peripherally (*black arrow*).

■ Differential Diagnosis

- ***Meniscal cyst:*** A cystic lesion that is hyperintense on T2-weighted images and abuts the meniscus in continuity with a meniscal tear is most likely a meniscal cyst.
- *Ganglion/synovial cyst:* This diagnosis is less likely given the adjacent meniscal tear and location of the cyst.
- *Atypical hemangioma:* The uniform hyperintense and homogeneous signal characteristics are not features of hemangiomas.

■ Essential Facts

- Meniscal cysts are commonly seen on MR examinations and may be lobulated or septate in appearance.
- The formation of a meniscal cyst is thought to be related to the extension of fluid through a meniscal tear.
- Direct communication between the meniscal cyst and the meniscal tear is common.
- Lateral meniscal cysts more often present as palpable masses, likely because of the relatively thin overlying lateral soft tissues.
- The treatment of a meniscal cyst involves decompression of the cyst and repair or resection of the tear.

✔ Pearls & ✘ Pitfalls

- ✔ Meniscal cysts are associated with horizontal cleavage tears and are more common medially.
- ✘ These cysts can be overlooked at arthroscopy because of their location.

Case 6

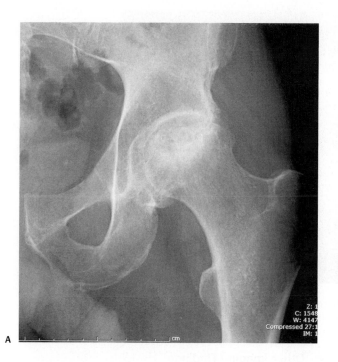 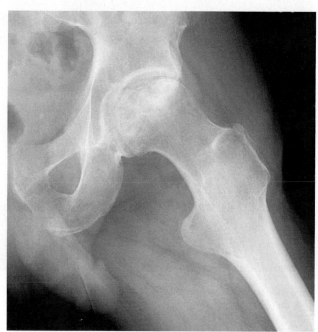

A

B

Clinical Presentation

The patient is a 52-year-old man with atraumatic pain in his left hip.

■ Imaging Findings

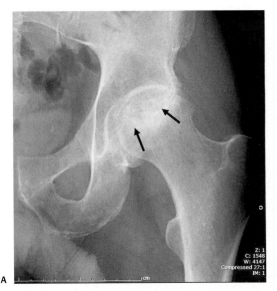 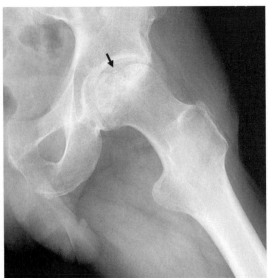

(A,B) Frontal and lateral radiographs of the left hip show patchy sclerosis (*long arrows*) involving the femoral head with superior articular collapse (*short arrow*). Joint space narrowing is present with a normal-appearing acetabulum.

■ Differential Diagnosis

- **Avascular necrosis (AVN):** Patchy sclerosis localized to the superior articular surface of the femoral head with focal articular collapse and a normal-appearing acetabulum is typical for AVN.
- *Osteoarthritis (OA):* The normal-appearing acetabulum and the unilaterality are atypical for OA.
- *Rheumatoid arthritis:* The pattern of joint space loss and the sclerotic changes are not features of this disease.

■ Essential Facts

- AVN is related to interruption of the blood supply with eventual infarction of the bone marrow.
- This process leads to articular collapse and can progress to secondary OA.
- The numerous causes include trauma, hemoglobinopathies, steroids, and alcoholism.
- A multitude of classification schemes exist for grading the severity.

■ Other Imaging Findings

- AVN may be detected with magnetic resonance imaging when the "double-line" sign is seen on T2-weighted sequences.

✔ Pearls & ✘ Pitfalls

- ✔ AVN typically originates as a unilateral process with sclerotic changes localized to the femoral head.
- ✘ Advanced AVN is difficult to diagnose as a result of secondary superimposed OA changes.

Case 7

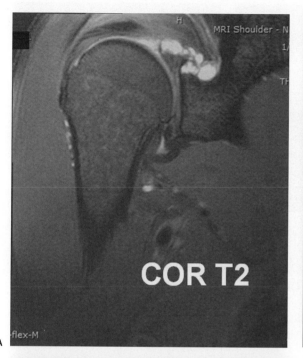

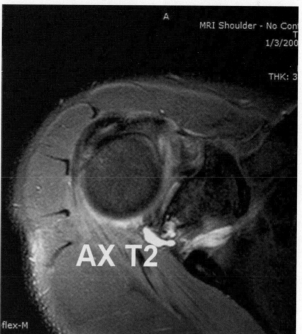

A

B

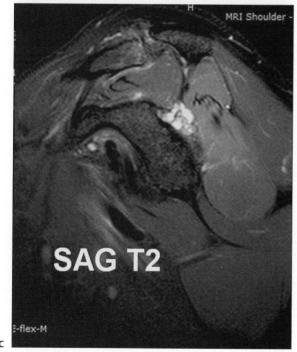

C

Clinical Presentation

The patient has chronic shoulder pain.

■ Imaging Findings

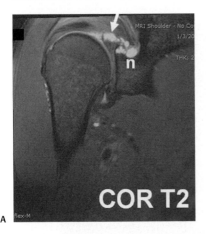
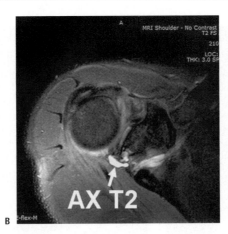
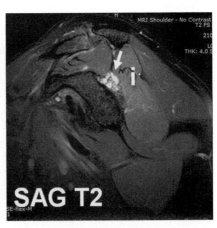

(A–C) Coronal, axial, and sagittal T2-weighted images show a cystic lesion (*arrows*) abutting the superior and posterior labral margin at the level of the spinoglenoid notch (n). Edema is present within the infraspinatus muscle (i).

■ Differential Diagnosis

• **Labral cyst:** T2-weighted magnetic resonance imaging (MRI) showing cystic changes approximating the glenoid labrum are most consistent with this diagnosis.

■ Essential Facts

• Labral cysts are associated with labral tears and represent the sequestration of joint fluid through the labral tear into the perilabral soft tissues.
• They may be associated with glenohumeral instability or may be incidentally noted on MRI.
• If present in the suprascapular or spinoglenoid notches, entrapment neuropathy of the suprascapular nerve may develop.

■ Other Imaging Findings

• MR arthrography may be performed to further characterize labral tears/cysts.

✔ Pearls & ✘ Pitfalls

✔ Labral cysts coexist with labral tears.
✘ Anterior labral cysts can be confused with fluid in the subscapular recess.

Case 8

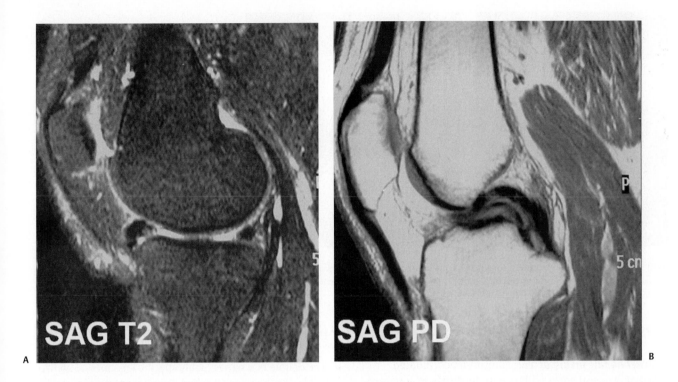

SAG T2

SAG PD

A

B

■ Clinical Presentation

The patient is a young adult with a locking knee.

■ Imaging Findings

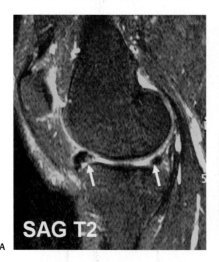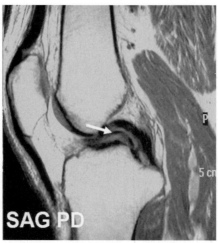

(A,B) Sagittal T2-weighted magnetic resonance (MR) images show blunting of the anterior and posterior horns (*arrows*) of the medial meniscus. A centrally displaced meniscal fragment causes a "double posterior cruciate ligament (PCL)" sign (*arrow*) on the proton density image.

■ Differential Diagnosis

• **Bucket handle meniscal tear:** Foreshortened, blunted medial meniscal horns with a centrally displaced fragment anterior and parallel to the PCL are characteristic findings of this lesion.

■ Essential Facts

• A bucket handle meniscal tear is an unstable tear; it is two times more common in the medial meniscus.
• This is a displaced, propagated, vertical tear; arthroscopy is required for attachment or removal of the fragment.
• The patient presents with locking of the knee.
• The name is derived from the central fragment, which resembles a handle, and the blunted peripheral meniscus, which resembles a bucket.

✔ Pearls & ✘ Pitfalls

✔ The double PCL sign is highly specific for a medial meniscus bucket handle tear when an intact anterior cruciate ligament and blunted medial meniscal horns are seen.
✘ The double PCL sign can be absent in up to 50% of cases, with the meniscal fragment displaced over the native anterior or posterior horn.

Case 9

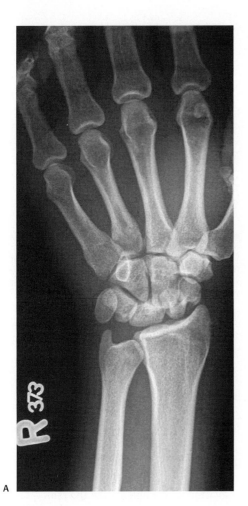 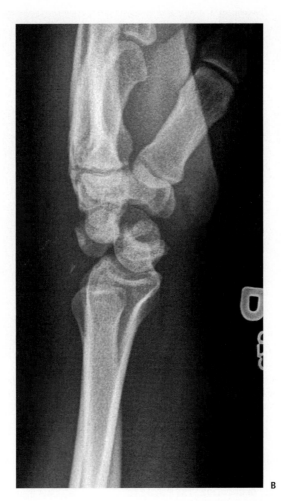

▪ Clinical Presentation

The patient has fallen onto an outstretched hand.

■ Imaging Findings

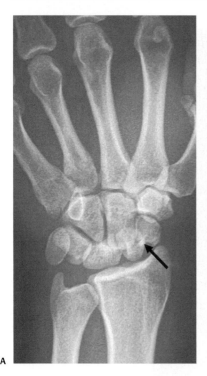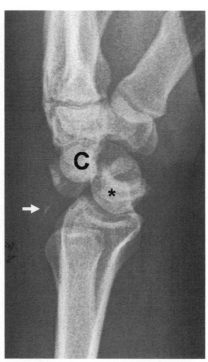

A   B

(A,B) Frontal and lateral views of the wrist show dorsal dislocation of the capitate bone (*C*) relative to the lunate bone (*asterisk*). The lunate bone remains in gross alignment with the radial articular surface. A fracture extends through the scaphoid bone (*long arrow*). Avulsion fragments over the dorsum of the wrist (*short arrow*) are related to the scaphoid fracture.

■ Differential Diagnosis

- ***Trans-scaphoid perilunate dislocation:*** The lunate remains aligned with the distal radius while the carpus is dorsally displaced and the scaphoid is fractured.

■ Essential Facts

- Trans-scaphoid perilunate dislocation results from a fall onto a hyperextended hand.
- The distal fragment of the scaphoid may move with the distal row of carpal bones.
- This is the second stage of progressive perilunate instability.

✔ Pearls & ✗ Pitfalls

- ✔ This injury is associated with scapholunate and radiocapitate ligament tears.
- ✗ The complex can be difficult to diagnose if the fracture fragments are markedly rotated and/or displaced.

Case 10

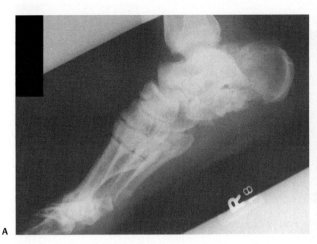

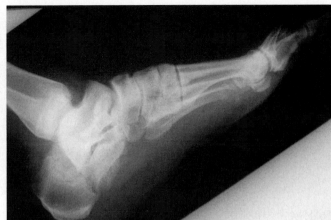

A   B

▨ Clinical Presentation
....

The patient has sustained a fall.

Further Work-up

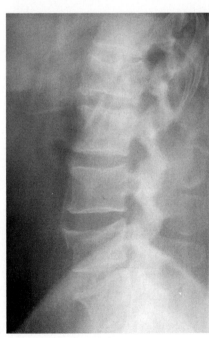

C

■ **Imaging Findings**

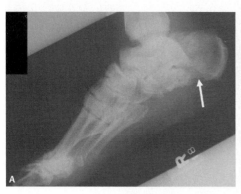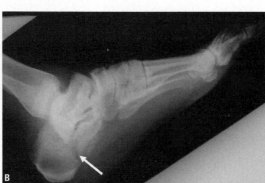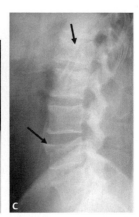

(A,B) Lateral views of both feet demonstrate highly comminuted, depressed intra-articular calcaneal fractures bilaterally (*arrows*). (C) Lateral view of the spine shows end plate compression fractures (*arrows*) at L1 and L4.

■ **Differential Diagnosis**

• ***Lover's fracture:*** Bilateral depressed intra-articular calcaneal fractures with associated compression fractures of the lumbar spine are characteristic of this entity.

■ **Essential Facts**

• Lover's fractures are intra-articular calcaneal fractures, 10% of which are bilateral.
• These calcaneal fractures result from an axial load and are associated with thoracolumbar fractures. Spinal radiographs are essential.
• Such calcaneal fractures typically have a poor prognosis because of displaced fragments.

✔ **Pearls & ✗ Pitfalls**

✔ Calcaneal fractures should alert the radiologist to evaluate for fractures of the thoracic and lumbar spine.
✗ The clinical presentation of the hindfoot fracture deformities may overshadow that of the spinal fractures.

Case 11

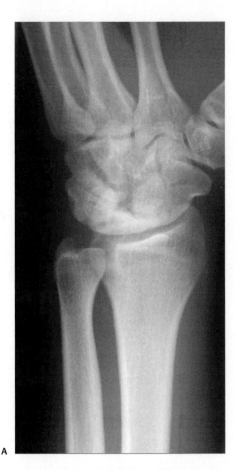 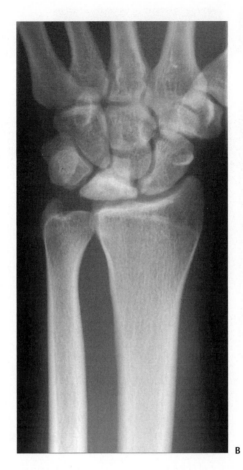

A   B

■ Clinical Presentation

The patient is a 30-year-old man with chronic wrist pain.

■ Imaging Findings

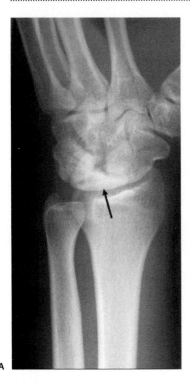 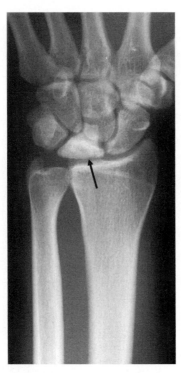

(A,B) Two views of the wrist demonstrate sclerosis and flattening of the lunate bone (*arrows*).

■ Differential Diagnosis

- ***Kienbock's disease:*** Increased density of the lunate bone relative to the other carpal bones and partial lunate collapse are distinctive findings in this disease process.

■ Essential Facts

- Kienbock's disease is a form of osteonecrosis.
- It is seen more commonly in manual laborers and in men between 20 and 40 years of age. The process causes progressive pain and swelling of the wrist.
- In approximately 75% of cases, the disease is associated with ulnar minus variance secondary to microtrauma resulting from uneven transfer of the carpal load across the lunate.

✔ Pearls & ✗ Pitfalls

- ✔ The process is more common on the right side and is rare in persons younger than 15 years of age.
- ✗ Typically, this entity cannot be detected on plain radiographs until it is in advanced stages.

Case 12

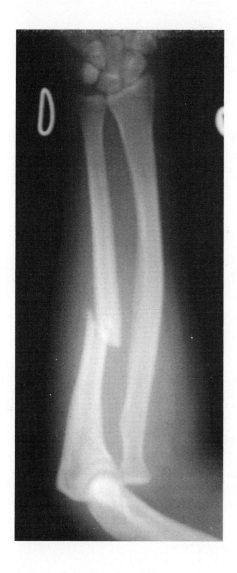

▧ Clinical Presentation

After a fall onto an outstretched hand, a patient presents with forearm pain.

◼ Imaging Findings

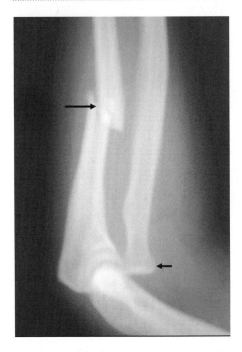

Lateral view of the forearm demonstrates a spiral fracture of the proximal ulnar diaphysis with anterior angulation of the apex (*long arrow*) and anterior dislocation of the radial head (*short arrow*).

◼ Differential Diagnosis

- **Monteggia fracture/dislocation:** This is a fracture of the proximal ulna with an associated dislocation of the radial head.

◼ Essential Facts

- Monteggia fracture/dislocation results from a fall onto an outstretched hand.
- Fractures of the ulna are usually proximal, and dislocations of the radial head are usually anterior.
- There is disruption of the proximal radioulnar joint and collateral ligaments of the elbow.
- Monteggia fracture/dislocation is rare in children.

✔ Pearls & ✘ Pitfalls

- ✔ The dislocation of the radial head follows the direction of angulation of the ulnar fracture.
- ✘ Dislocations of the radial head may be overlooked in children.

Case 13

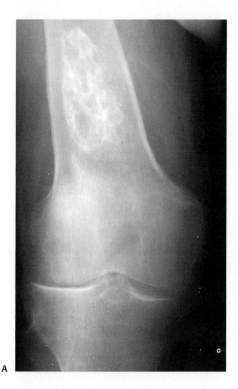

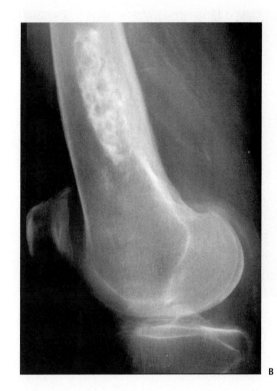

A

B

■ Clinical Presentation

An abnormality of the knee is seen on outside radiographs.

Further Work-up

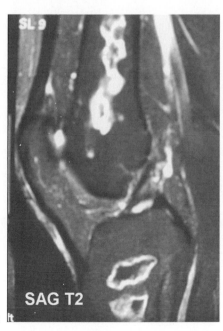

SL 9

SAG T2

C

■ Imaging Findings

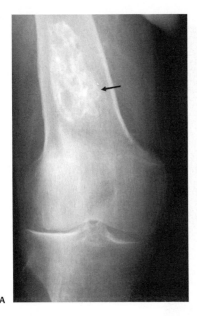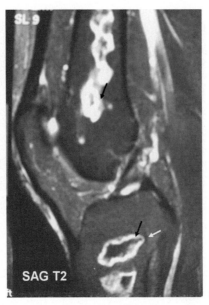

A   B

(A) Radiograph of the knee displays serpentine sclerosis with a lobular appearance (*arrow*) in the distal femoral diametaphyseal medullary canal. **(B)** T2-weighted sagittal image demonstrates geographic, abnormal changes of increased T2 signal intensity (*black arrows*) in the femur and tibia. A low-signal border (*white arrow*) outlines the increased T2 signal in the tibia. These combined alterations in the T2 signal represent the "double-line" sign.

■ Differential Diagnosis

- **Bone infarct/osteonecrosis:** Circumscribed lobular/serpentine sclerotic changes in the medulla canal on plain radiographs with features of a double-line sign on T2-weighted magnetic resonance imaging (MRI) are diagnostic.
- *Enchondroma:* The pattern of chondroid mineralization and lobular T2 signal changes are absent in this case.

■ Essential Facts

- Osteonecrosis, or bone infarct, is ischemic death in the bone marrow with a multitude of causes, including steroids, hemoglobinopathies, renal transplant, and pancreatitis.
- The process is identical to avascular necrosis except that it does not involve an articular surface.
- On MRI, the high T2 signal intensity represents cellular regenerative changes. The peripheral rim of low T2 signal intensity represents serpentine sclerosis, which can be seen on plain radiographs.
- These findings are collectively referred to as the double-line sign.
- Clinical manifestations can include localized bone pain and soft-tissue swelling.
- Rare malignant degeneration can be seen.

✔ Pearls & ✘ Pitfalls

- ✔ Bone infarcts are common in the diametaphyseal regions of long bones with a high fat content.
- ✘ Radiographic findings are negative in the early stages of this process.

Case 14

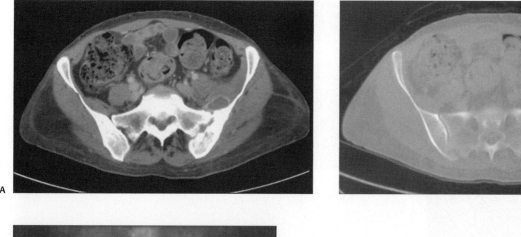

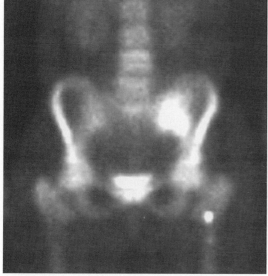

■ Clinical Presentation

The patient is a 40-year-old woman with polysubstance abuse and severe low back pain.

■ Imaging Findings

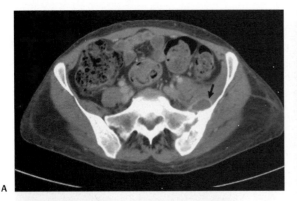

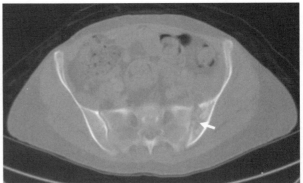

A

B

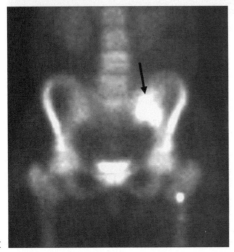

C

(A–C) Axial computed tomographic scan through the sacroiliac (SI) joints shows extensive erosion of the left SI joint (A, *white arrow*) with an anterior rim-enhancing fluid collection (B, *black arrow*). Radionuclide examination shows increased uptake over the left SI joint (C, *arrow*).

■ Differential Diagnosis

- ***Infectious sacroiliitis:*** The combination of the clinical history and asymmetric destructive erosions of the SI joint with an adjacent abscess is pathognomonic for this process.
- *Seronegative spondyloarthropathy:* The clinical presentation and adjacent rim-enhancing fluid collection are not representative of this disease class.
- *Metastasis:* An articular destructive process with inflammatory findings in the adjacent soft tissue does not favor neoplasia.

■ Essential Facts

- Infectious sacroiliitis may be related to contiguous spread from an adjacent infection (e.g., decubitus ulcers), to hematogenous spread from the intestines or genitourinary tract via Batson's plexus, or to intravenous drug abuse.
- Staphylococci and streptococci are the typical offending organisms.
- A destructive, poorly marginated lesion of the SI joint associated with soft-tissue swelling is often seen.
- Abscess formation within the presacral soft tissues is not uncommon.

■ Other Imaging Findings

- MRI is ideal for early detection showing decreased T1 and increased T2 signal replacing the normal marrow of the involved SI joint.

✔ Pearls & ✗ Pitfalls

- ✔ SI joint infection is typically unilateral, with destruction of the subchondral bone that is usually more extensive on the iliac side of the articulation.
- ✗ Radiography is insensitive early in the disease process.

Case 15

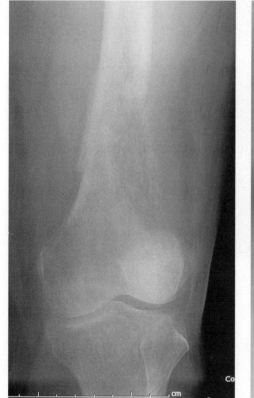
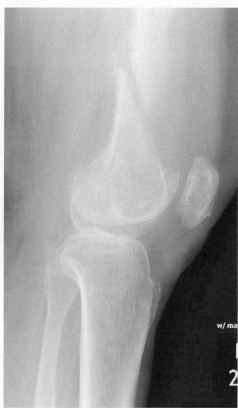

A

B

■ Clinical Presentation

The 53-year-old patient has experienced a fall.

■ Imaging Findings

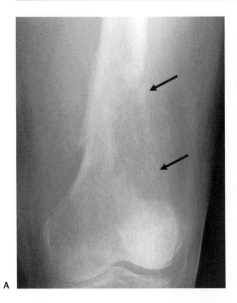 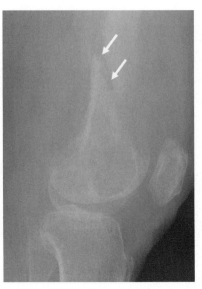

A   B

(A,B) Radiographs of the knee display a spiral fracture (B, *white arrows*) coursing through an ill-defined, eccentric lytic/permeative lesion (A, *black arrows*) involving the distal femoral corticomedullary junction.

■ Differential Diagnosis

• ***Pathologic fracture (metastatic bronchogenic carcinoma):*** A lytic lesion superimposed on a spiral fracture is characteristic of this diagnosis.

■ Essential Facts

• Metastasis to bone is the most common malignant bone tumor in adults, and a pathologic fracture may be the first clinical manifestation of this process.
• Up to 40% of cases of metastatic bronchogenic carcinoma involve the skeleton.
• Hematogenous spread is the typical route, with medullary, cortical, or subcortical invasion.
• The extent of cortical bone destruction is correlated with the likelihood of a pathologic fracture.

✔ Pearls & ✘ Pitfalls

✔ Metastases of bronchogenic carcinoma tend to affect the appendicular skeleton distal to the knees and elbows.
✘ Subacute healing of a nonpathologic fracture may mimic a pathologic fracture.

Case 16

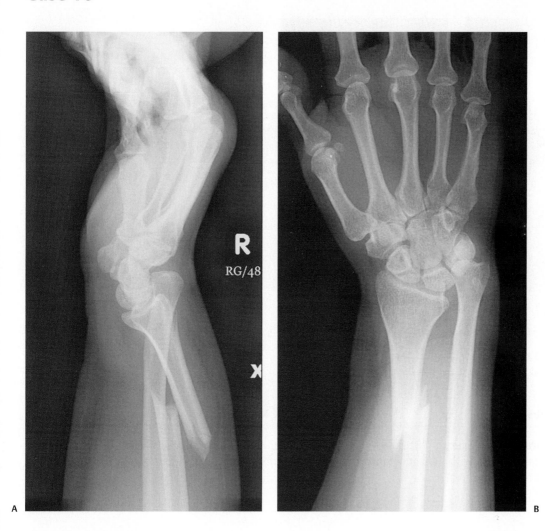

Clinical Presentation

After trauma, a patient presents with deformity of the right wrist.

■ Imaging Findings

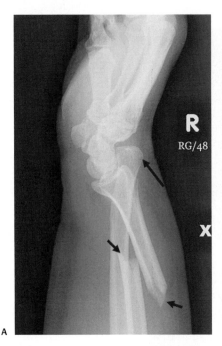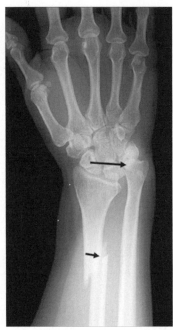

(A,B) Radiographs of the wrist demonstrate an overriding spiral fracture of the distal radius (*short arrows*) in conjunction with a dorsally dislocated ulna (*long arrow*).

■ Differential Diagnosis

• *Galeazzi fracture/dislocation:* This injury is a fracture involving the distal radial diaphysis with subsequent ulnar dislocation at the distal radial–ulnar joint.

■ Essential Facts

• A Galeazzi fracture/dislocation results from a fall onto an outstretched hand with a pronated forearm.
• The fracture extends through the distal radius with disruption of the distal radial–ulnar joint.
• This injury can be complicated, with a delayed union or nonunion of the radial fracture or entrapment of the extensor carpi ulnaris tendon.

✔ Pearls & ✘ Pitfalls

✔ The ulnar dislocations are typically dorsal.
✘ Subtle dorsal ulnar subluxations may be missed if a true lateral radiograph is not provided.

Case 17

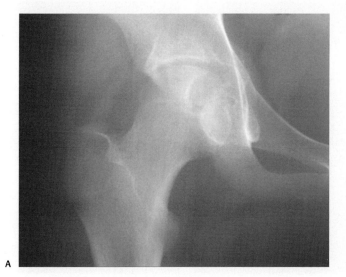

A

Clinical Presentation

The patient is 15-year-old girl with chronic pain in the right hip.

Further Work-up

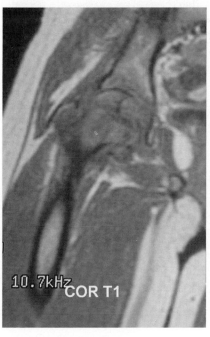

B

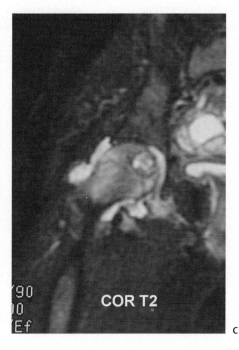

C

■ Imaging Findings

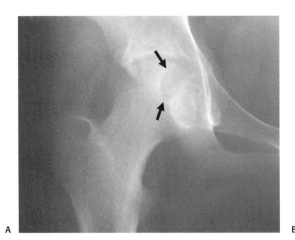
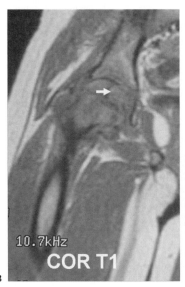
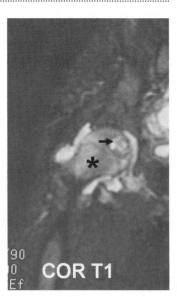

(A) A frontal radiograph of the right hip displays a nonmineralized lytic lesion with a sclerotic rim centered in the femoral epiphysis (*arrows*). **(B,C)** Coronal T1- and T2-weighted magnetic resonance imaging (MRI) shows an intermediate T1 signal and heterogeneous intermediate T2 signal within the lesion (*arrows*) with extensive marrow edema (*asterisk*) and a joint effusion.

■ Differential Diagnosis

- **Chondroblastoma:** A circumscribed osteolytic lesion of the epiphysis with a sclerotic rim is a common radiographic feature. Lobulated heterogeneous intermediate T2 signal intensity and surrounding edema are fairly distinctive MRI features.
- *Eosinophilic granuloma/Brodie's abscess:* Heterogeneous intermediate T2 signal intensity with extensive surrounding bony edema is atypical for this lesion.

■ Essential Facts

- Chondroblastoma is a benign cartilaginous neoplasm common in the second and third decades of life.
- It is more prevalent in boys.
- Patients present with pain and swelling.
- The lesions arise in the epiphyses of long bones, most commonly the tibia, femur, and humerus.
- A calcified chondroid matrix is seen in 30 to 50% of chondroblastomas.

✔ Pearls & ✗ Pitfalls

- ✔ A high percentage (60%) show low-to-intermediate T2 signal intensity within the cartilage matrix with severe surrounding edema.
- ✗ Up to 15% may show fluid–fluid levels on MRI, causing confusion with aneurysmal bone cysts.

Case 18

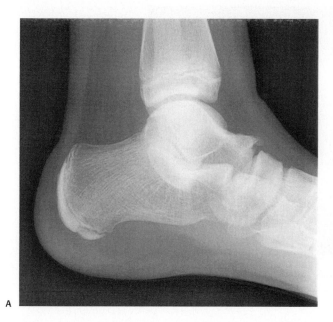

A

■ Clinical Presentation

A 15-year-old boy has chronic midfoot pain.

Further Work-up

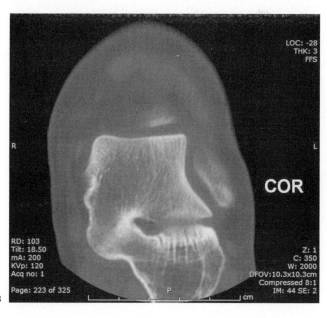

B

■ Imaging Findings

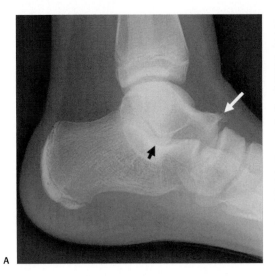 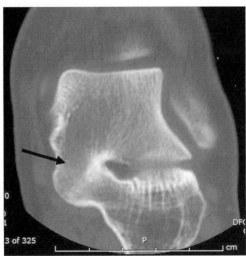

(A) Lateral ankle radiograph demonstrates a talar beak (*white arrow*) with absence of the middle facet of the subtalar joint (*black arrow*). (B) Coronal computed tomographic (CT) scan shows osseous fusion across the middle facet (*arrow*) of the subtalar joint.

■ Differential Diagnosis

• **Talocalcaneal coalition:** Radiographic talar beaking with absence of the middle facet and CT demonstration of osseous fusion across the middle facet are distinct features of this diagnosis.

■ Essential Facts

• Tarsal talocalcaneal coalition is thought to be congenitally related to abnormal segmentation of the tarsal bones.
• This process may be osseous, fibrous, or cartilaginous.
• Patients may present with peroneal spastic flatfoot.
• This is the second most common coalition after calcaneonavicular coalition.
• A talar beak develops secondary to abnormal motion through the subtalar joint.

✔ Pearls & ✗ Pitfalls

✔ Tarsal coalition is bilateral in approximately 50% of cases.
✗ This process can be difficult to visualize on radiographic views because of the complex orientation of the subtalar joint.

Case 19

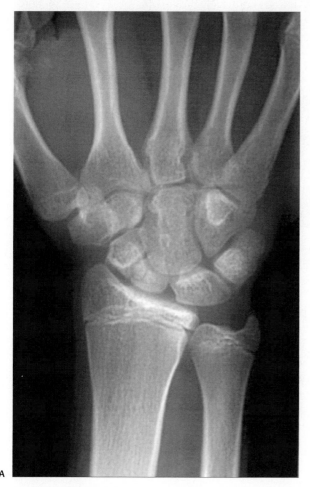

A

▪ Clinical Presentation

Patient with remote history of trauma with snuff box tenderness.

Further Work-up

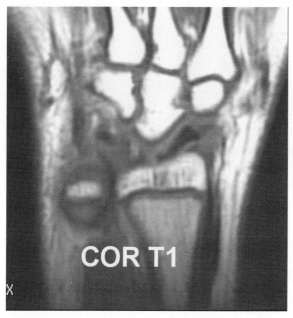

B

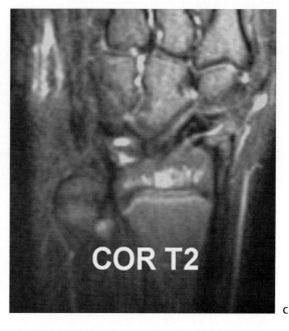

C

■ Imaging Findings

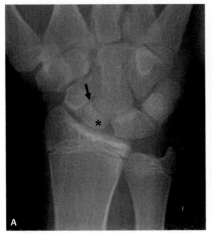 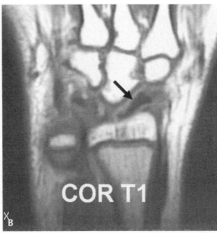 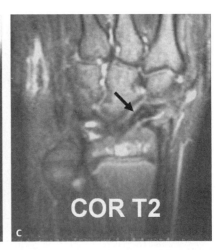

(A) Radiograph of the wrist show a subacute fracture line (*arrow*) interrupting the waist of the scaphoid bone with sclerotic change involving the proximal pole fragment (*asterisk*). **(B,C)** Magnetic resonance imaging (MRI) displays persistent decreased signal intensity through the proximal pole fragment (*arrows*), indicating necrotic bone.

■ Differential Diagnosis

- **Subacute scaphoid waist fracture with osteonecrosis:**
  Plain radiographs demonstrate a scaphoid waist fracture without gross displacement. Sclerosis of the proximal fragment correlating with MRI findings of low signal intensity on T1- and T2-weighted images represents osteonecrosis.

■ Essential Facts

- The scaphoid is the most commonly fractured carpal bone.
- Scaphoid fracture is caused by a fall onto an outstretched hand.
- More distal fractures have a better prognosis.
- Osteonecrosis occurs with fractures through the proximal pole/waist, which disrupt the distal-to-proximal blood flow.
- Osteonecrosis develops after 10 to 15% of scaphoid injuries. It may take 4 to 8 weeks for radiographic changes of sclerosis to develop.

✔ Pearls & ✘ Pitfalls

- ✔ Seventy percent of scaphoid fractures occur through the waist.
- ✘ Rarely, scaphoid osteonecrosis may develop in the absence of prior trauma; this condition is referred to as Preiser's disease.

Case 20

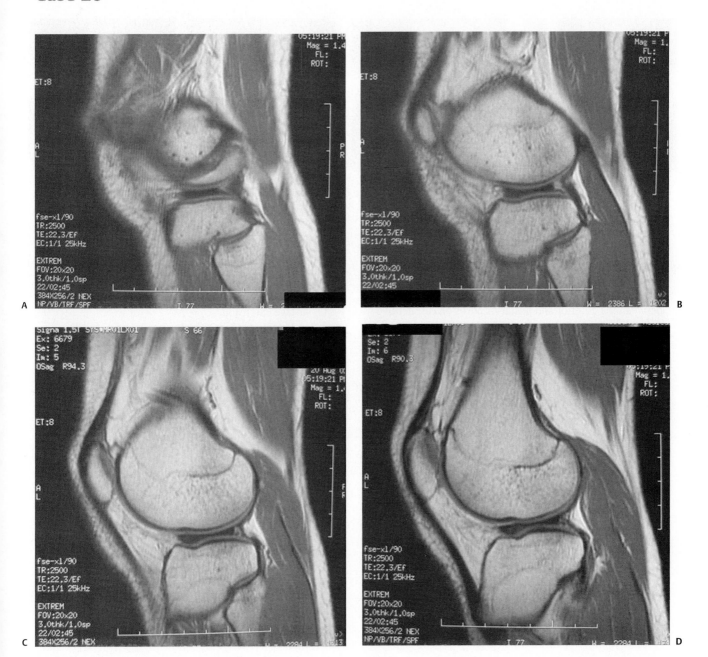

■ Clinical Presentation

A 15-year-old girl presents with pain and snapping of the knee.

■ Imaging Findings

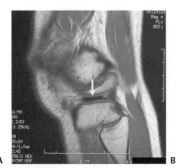 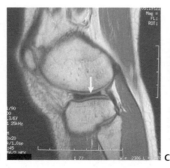 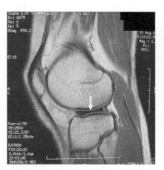 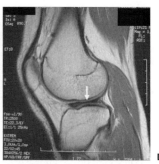

A   B   C   D

(A–D) Sagittal magnetic resonance images of the knee through the lateral compartment show an abnormally thickened, broad, disklike lateral meniscus (*arrows*) with continuous meniscal tissue bridging the anterior and posterior horns.

■ Differential Diagnosis

- **Discoid meniscus:** The abnormal discoid appearance of the lateral meniscus with continuation of meniscal tissue between the anterior and posterior horns on consecutive sagittal images is characteristic of this diagnosis.

■ Essential Facts

- The diagnosis of a discoid meniscus is suggested by the identification of either meniscal tissue on three continuous sagittal 5-mm-thick slices or a meniscal body on coronal images > 15 mm wide or extending into the intercondylar notch.
- The end result is redundant meniscal tissue covering a large portion of the femoral–tibial articular surface.
- Discoid menisci are more common laterally. No unified theory exists on the etiology or classification.

✔ Pearls & ✘ Pitfalls

- ✔ A symptomatic knee with abnormal signal within this meniscal variant is considered a tear, regardless of articular surface extension.
- ✘ A nondisplaced tear of this meniscal variant may be confused with a bucket handle tear.

Case 21

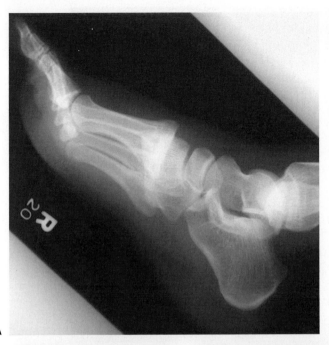

A

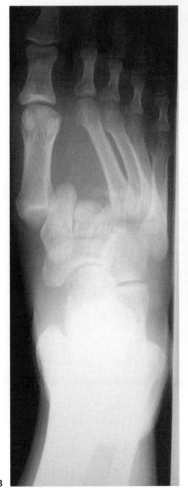

B

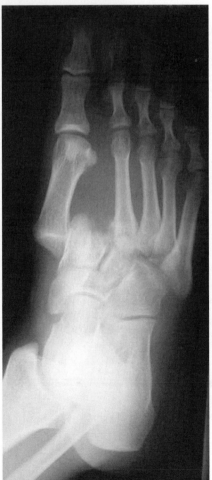

C

■ Clinical Presentation

Patient with foot pain following motor vehicle collision.

■ Imaging Findings

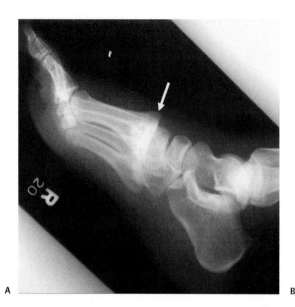
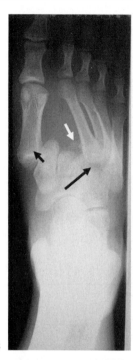
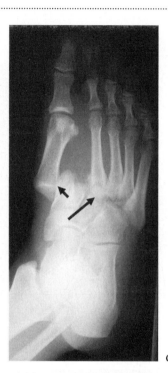

A   B   C

(A–C) Multiple views of the foot show dorsal subluxation of the metatarsal (MT) bases on the lateral view (**A,** *long white arrow*). Lateral dislocation of the second through fourth tarsometatarsal (TMT) joints (**B,C,** *long black arrow*) and medial dislocation of the first TMT joint (**B,C,** *short black arrow*) are seen. Bony fragments project in the first intermetatarsal space (**B,** *short white arrow*).

■ Differential Diagnosis

- ***Divergent Lisfranc fracture/dislocation:*** The patient's presentation and the divergent pattern of dislocation across the TMT joints are distinct for this injury.
- *Charcot joint:* Although divergent Lisfranc fracture/dislocation is common with Charcot joint, the cardinal features of chronic fragmentation, sclerosis, debris, and vascular calcifications are lacking.

■ Essential Facts

- This injury results when a violent abduction to a fixed forefoot causes distraction of the Lisfranc ligament, which anchors the second MT base to the medial cuneiform bone.
- The injury leads to either a homolateral (first MT base dislocates laterally) or divergent (first MT base dislocates medially) dislocation across the TMT junction.
- The second through fourth MT bases typically dislocate dorsally and laterally. However, subtle subluxation at the second TMT joint may be the only manifestation. These injuries must be surgically corrected.

■ Other Imaging Findings

- Magnetic resonance imaging may be used to evaluate the Lisfranc ligament.

✔ Pearls & ✗ Pitfalls

- ✔ This injury should be suspected when offset is noted between the medial margin of the second MT and the medial margin of the intermediate cuneiform bone at the level of the second TMT joint.
- ✗ Occasionally, forefoot malalignment may not be evident unless stress views are obtained.

Case 22

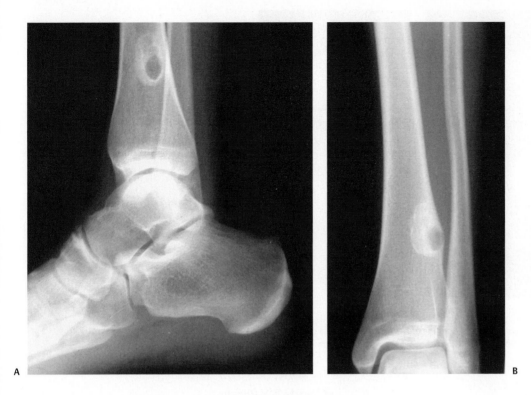

A   B

◼ Clinical Presentation

A 16-year-old patient presents with a sprained ankle.

■ Imaging Findings

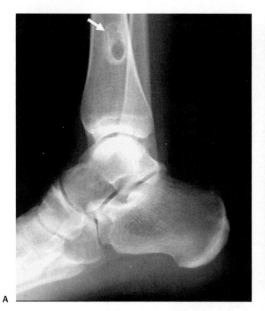
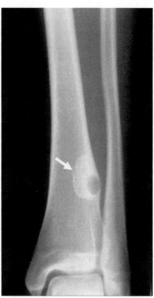

A   B

(A,B) Images of the ankle show a circumscribed, rounded area of lucency based in the medial tibial cortex and enclosed by a thick, organized rim of sclerosis (*arrows*). The process causes a smooth contour abnormality of the medial tibial cortex without periostitis or a soft-tissue mass.

■ Differential Diagnosis

- ***Nonossifying fibroma:*** The location, patient's age, and radiographic characteristics are classic for this diagnosis.
- *Osteoid osteoma:* A smaller radiolucent nidus with surrounding periostitis is characteristic of this lesion.
- *Brodie abscess:* Disorganized sclerosis and periostitis are typically seen with this process.

■ Essential Facts

- Nonossifying fibroma is a benign cortex-based tumor seen in children older than 2 years of age. It is rare in adults.
- The development of this lesion is thought to be related to trauma at the attachment of a muscle to a long bone, with the femur and tibia the most common sites of involvement.
- The lesion involutes and is eventually replaced by normal bone.
- Nonossifying fibromas are painless and often detected incidentally.

✔ Pearls & ✘ Pitfalls

- ✔ This lesion is common along the posterior and medial aspects of the tibial and femoral cortices and is rare in children not yet walking. The process is uncommon in the upper extremities.
- ✘ When large and expansile, nonossifying fibromas may resemble aneurysmal bone cysts.

Case 23

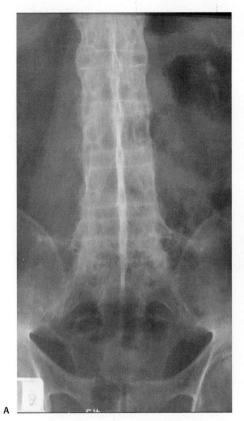 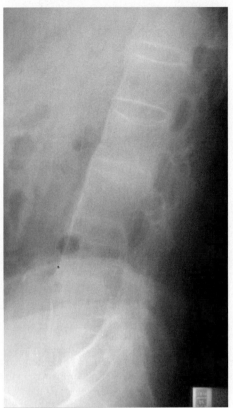

A   B

■ Clinical Presentation

A 40-year-old man presents with back stiffness.

■ Imaging Findings

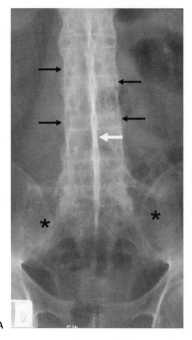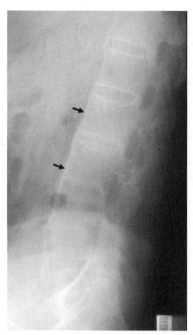

A   B

(A,B) Two views of the lumbar spine demonstrate bilateral sacroiliac (SI) joint fusion (*asterisks*). The lateral view displays squaring of the anterior lumbar vertebral body cortices (*short black arrows*), related to new bone formation. Syndesmophytes (*long black arrows*) bridge the vertebral bodies, causing the appearance of a "bamboo spine" on the frontal radiograph. Dense ossification of the interspinous ligament (*white arrow*) causes a "dagger" sign.

■ Differential Diagnosis

- ***Ankylosing spondylitis:*** Bilateral SI joint fusion with a "bamboo spine" in a young man with back pain is diagnostic.
- *Diffuse idiopathic skeletal hyperostosis (DISH):* This type of paravertebral ossification is bulkier and tends to occur in older individuals.
- *Psoriatic arthritis:* This process produces thick, irregular paravertebral ossification with asymmetric SI joint findings.

■ Essential Facts

- Ankylosing spondylitis is a chronic inflammatory arthritic condition common in young men between the ages of 15 and 35 years that primarily affects the axial skeleton, synovial/cartilaginous joints, and entheses.
- Erosive changes are followed by bone formation, with fusion typically affecting the SI joints and spine.
- Many patients are seropositive for HLA-B27, suggesting a hereditary component.

✔ Pearls & ✘ Pitfalls

- ✔ SI joint involvement must be present to make the diagnosis. Syndesmophyte formation originates at the thoracolumbar junction.
- ✘ The radiographic appearance can be identical to skeletal changes caused by inflammatory bowel disease (e.g., Crohn's disease).

Case 24

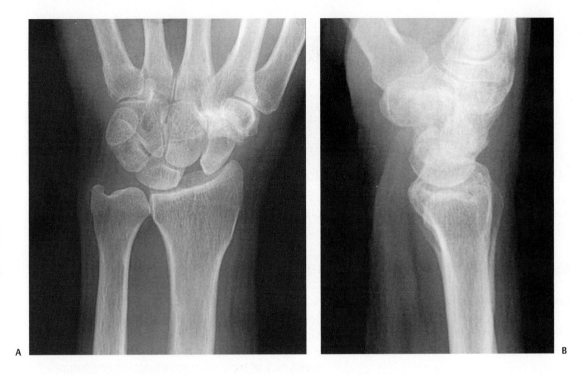

A B

▪ Clinical Presentation

The patient presents with chronic wrist pain and a remote history of trauma.

Further Work-up

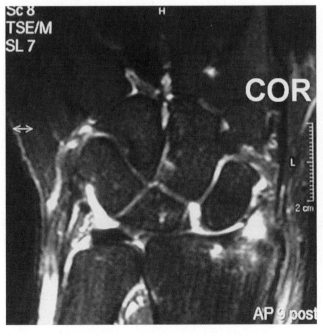

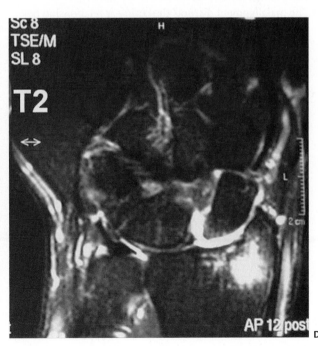

C D

■ Imaging Findings

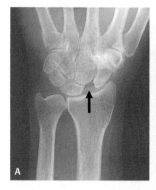 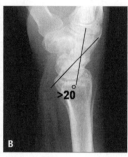 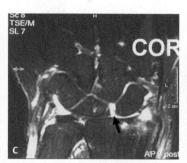 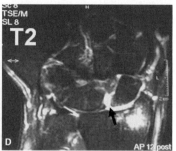

(A,B) Radiographs of the wrist show abnormal widening (*arrow*) between the scaphoid and lunate bones. The lateral view shows loss of the co-linear relationship between the capitate and lunate bones (normal variation, < 20 degrees). (C,D) Coronal T2-weighted magnetic resonance images of the wrist demonstrate absence of the scapholunate ligament (*arrows*).

■ Differential Diagnosis

• ***Scapholunate dissociation with dorsal intercalated segmental instability (DISI):*** The combined features of widening of the scapholunate interval with dorsal lunate tilt and absence of the scapholunate ligament are characteristic of this diagnosis.

■ Essential Facts

• Scapholunate dissociation with DISI is caused by a dorsiflexion injury.
• Disruption of the scapholunate ligament causes the lunate bone to flex toward the dorsum of the hand.
• The malalignment disrupts the co-linear relationship between the capitate and lunate bones, with widening of the scapholunate interval of > 5 mm on flexion of the scaphoid. This pattern is more common than its counterpart, volar intercalated segmental instability (VISI).
• The injury is part of a spectrum of abnormalities leading to perilunate dislocation.

✔ Pearls & ✗ Pitfalls

✔ Scapholunate dissociation with DISI commonly occurs after scaphoid fractures. Posteroanterior radiographs often show a flexed scaphoid with a "signet ring" appearance.
✗ Radiographic findings may be normal, and clenched fist views may be required to accentuate the scapholunate widening.

Case 25

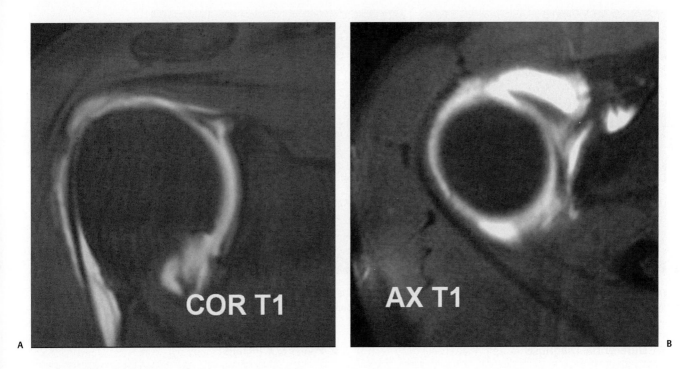

■ Clinical Presentation

A college baseball pitcher presents with shoulder pain.

■ Imaging Findings

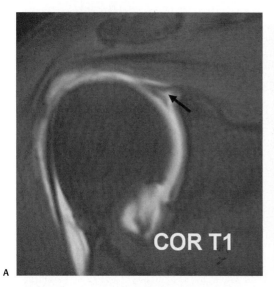
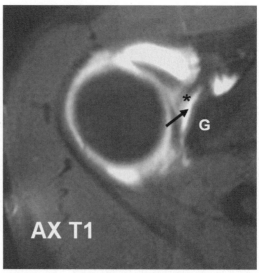

A   B

(A,B) Coronal image from a magnetic resonance (MR) arthrogram shows superior labral lateral undercutting (*arrow*); axial image demonstrates a defect (*arrow*) between the bony glenoid (*G*) and the superior labral margin (*asterisk*).

■ Differential Diagnosis

- **Superior labral anterior–posterior (SLAP) tear:** Intra-articular contrast extending into the superior labral anterior and posterior quadrants is characteristic of this lesion.
- *Sublabral recess:* This normal recess is typically not seen so far posteriorly along the superior aspect of the labrum. Additionally, it is oriented in a medial direction on coronal images.

■ Essential Facts

- The SLAP tear involves the superior labral quadrants and is related to repetitive overhead activity or falling on an outstretched arm.
- The biceps tendon is thought to place traction on the superior labrum, which causes eventual detachment from the glenoid fossa.
- Multiple types of SLAP lesions have been described. The lesion is best diagnosed with MR arthrography.

✔ Pearls & ✘ Pitfalls

- ✔ Lateral superior labral undercutting containing high T2 signal intensity or intra-articular contrast represents a labral tear.
- ✘ In the absence of joint fluid, these lesions may be undetectable.

Case 26

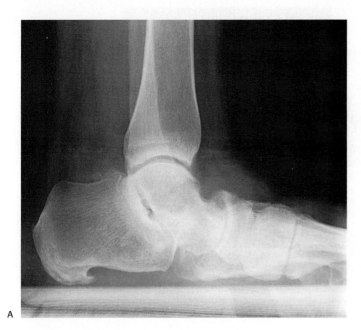

A

■ Clinical Presentation

A 55-year-old woman presents with progressive midfoot pain.

Further Work-up

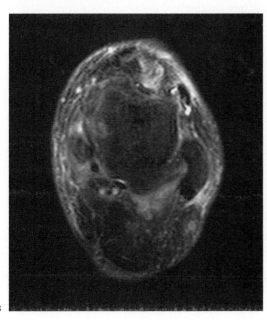

B

■ Imaging Findings

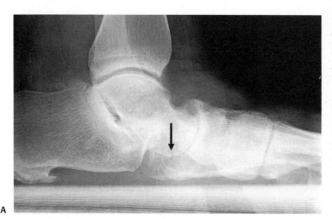
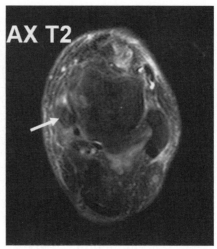

(A) A lateral weight-bearing view of the foot shows midfoot collapse with plantar subluxation of the talar head (*arrow*) relative to the navicular bone. (B) Axial T2-weighted magnetic resonance imaging (MRI) of the ankle shows enlargement of the posterior tibial tendon (*arrow*) with areas of increased T2 signal intensity.

■ Differential Diagnosis

- **Posterior tibial tendon tear:** Midfoot collapse on a lateral weight-bearing radiograph of the foot and posterior tibial tendon enlargement with interstitial T2 signal intensity increase on MRI are distinct features of a posterior tibial tendon tear.

■ Essential Facts

- Posterior tibial tendon tears are typically a chronic injury seen in women in the fifth and sixth decades of life.
- They are common in obese patients and those with inflammatory arthropathies.
- Patients present with a progressive flatfoot deformity that results in failure of the longitudinal arch.
- Posterior tibial tendon disease commonly coexists with spring ligament failure.
- Tears are common at the level of the medial malleolus secondary to friction from the 90-degree turn.
- Such tears may require surgical repair.

✔ Pearls & ✘ Pitfalls

- ✔ On axial MRI, the posterior tibial tendon should be no more than twice the size of the flexor digitorum tendon. Posterior tibial tenosynovitis may manifest as medial malleolar periostitis on plain radiographs.
- ✘ Non-weight-bearing radiographs of the feet may not reveal midfoot collapse.

Case 27

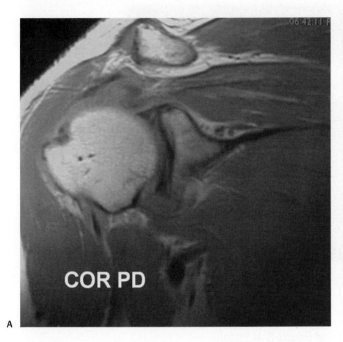

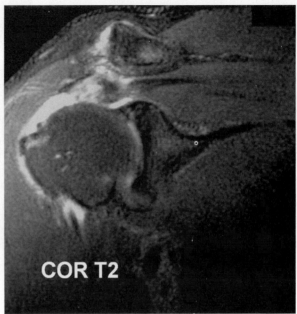

A B

■ Clinical Presentation

A 40-year-old man presents with acute shoulder pain and normal findings on radiographs.

■ Imaging Findings

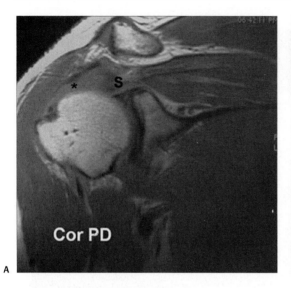 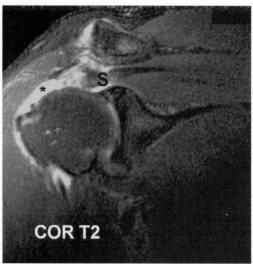

(A,B) Coronal images of the shoulder demonstrate complete discontinuity of the supraspinatus tendon (*S*). Retraction of the tendon creates a fluid-filled gap (*asterisk*).

■ Differential Diagnosis

- **Full-thickness rotator cuff tear:** Magnetic resonance imaging (MRI) findings of cranial–caudal tendon disruption extending to both the bursal and articular margins with tendon retraction creating a fluid-filled gap are consistent with a full-thickness tear.

■ Essential Facts

- Full-thickness tears of the rotator cuff, which are common in the athletic shoulder, result from impingement by the adjacent bony structures: the acromion, clavicle, humeral head, and glenoid fossa.
- The supraspinatus tendon is the most commonly involved structure. Initially, tendonosis develops in a hypovascular region termed the critical zone. If untreated, this condition may eventually lead to a tear.
- If untreated, this condition may eventually lead to a tear.
- The typical mechanism is tensile overuse related to overhead throwing. It is important to report the amount of tendon retraction and fatty atrophy, as this will affect management.

✔ Pearls & ✘ Pitfalls

- ✔ On frontal radiographs, a humeral head abutting the undersurface of the acromion is diagnostic of a full-thickness rotator cuff tear.
- ✘ Smaller, chronic full-thickness rotator cuff tears may be difficult to diagnose on MRI in the absence of a joint effusion or without intra-articular contrast.

Case 28

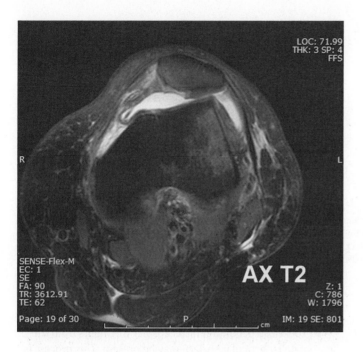

▨ Clinical Presentation

A 30-year-old woman presents with severe knee pain.

■ Imaging Findings

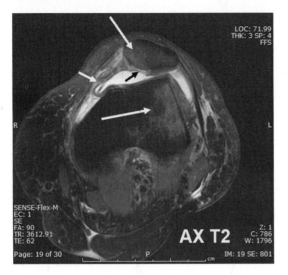

Axial T2-weighted image through the patellofemoral joint displays contusions over the periphery of the lateral condyle and medial patella (*long white arrows*). There is disruption of the medial patellofemoral retinaculum (*short white arrow*), with a chondral defect centered over the patellar apex (*short black arrow*). Lateral translation of the patella is present

■ Differential Diagnosis

• *Lateral patellofemoral dislocation:* Bone contusions over the lateral condyle and medial patellar facet are present. Disruption of the medial patellofemoral retinaculum allows lateral patellar translation. Chondral defects over the patellar apex and medial facet are also present. These are distinct features of lateral patellofemoral dislocation.

■ Essential Facts

• Dislocation of the patellofemoral joint is most often transient.
• Lateral dislocation predominates secondary to the sum lateral vector of forces related to the anatomy of the extensor mechanism.
• The process usually follows a twisting injury.
• The medial patellar facet impacts the lateral condyle, bruising bone and damaging the medial patellar facet cartilage.
• The medial patellofemoral retinaculum may rupture, causing the patient to present with medial joint line pain mimicking that of a medial meniscal tear.
• Magnetic resonance imaging (MRI) is the modality of choice for evaluating this injury.

✔ Pearls & ✘ Pitfalls

✔ Loose osteochondral intracapsular fragments from the patellar articular surface may be present. This process is more common in female patients.
✘ Patients typically do not report a history of patellar dislocation, and MRI findings may be subtle in the chronic stages. The findings on plain radiographs are often normal.

Case 29

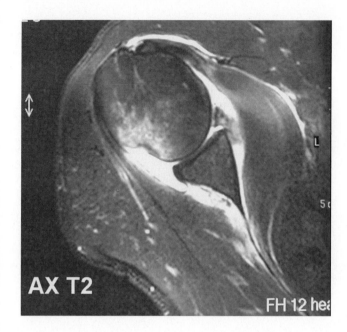

Clinical Presentation

A patient who has fallen presents with shoulder pain and normal radiographic findings.

■ Imaging Findings

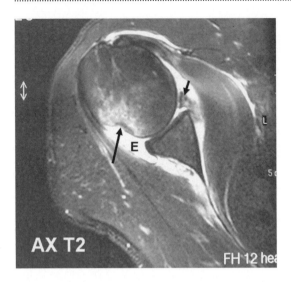

Axial T2-weighted images through the glenohumeral joint show an effusion (*E*). An impaction fracture with edema (*long arrow*) overlies the posterolateral humeral head with detachment of the anterior labrum (*short arrow*).

■ Differential Diagnosis

• **Hill–Sachs lesion/cartilaginous Bankart lesion from anterior shoulder dislocation:** An impaction fracture through the posterolateral humeral head (Hill–Sachs lesion) in conjunction with an anterior labral tear (cartilaginous Bankart lesion) is diagnostic of prior anterior glenohumeral joint dislocation.

■ Essential Facts

• Anterior shoulder dislocations represent 95% of all shoulder dislocations.
• These injuries are associated with impaction fractures of the posterolateral humeral head (Hill–Sachs lesion), which is driven against the anterior rim of the glenoid fossa, causing a bony (Bankart fracture) or cartilaginous (Bankart lesion) glenoid defect.
• This injury often results from an abrupt abduction and external rotation force.
• Recurrence rates are high in patients with a first-time dislocation who are younger than 30 years of age. Magnetic resonance (MR) arthrography is the ideal examination for evaluating this injury.

✔ Pearls & ✘ Pitfalls

✔ A Hill–Sachs lesion is most reliably diagnosed on the three proximal most axial images through the humeral head on conventional MR imaging.
✘ Findings on plain radiographs often appear normal.

Case 30

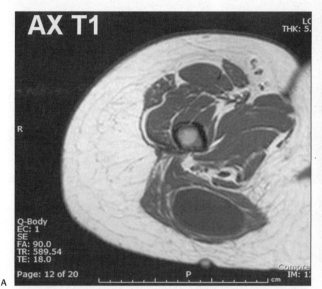

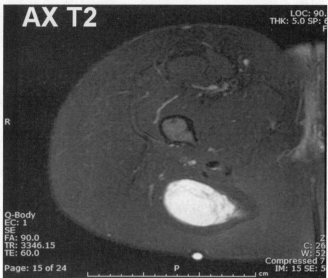

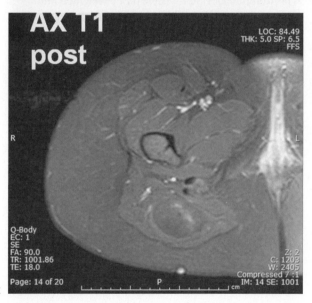

Clinical Presentation

A 27-year-old woman presents with a buttock mass.

■ Imaging Findings

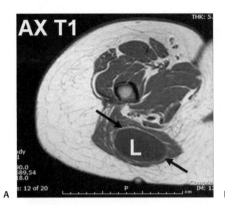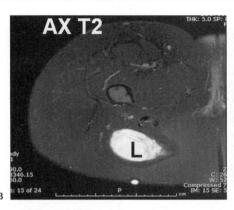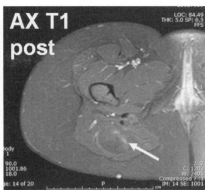

A   B   C

(A–C) A well-defined intragluteal ovoid lesion (*L*) with fluidlike signal intensity appears on axial T1- and T2-weighted magnetic resonance (MR) images. A peritumoral fat rind is visible on the T1-weighted MR image (*black arrows*). Whorled internal enhancement (*white arrow*) is seen.

■ Differential Diagnosis

- ***Intramuscular myxoma:*** A solitary, circumscribed intramuscular lesion with fluidlike signal intensity and internal enhancement is likely a myxoma.
- *Myxoid liposarcoma:* The absence of fatty nodules and/or fatty septa argues against this lesion.
- *Hematoma:* Typically, this process will show heterogeneity on MR images, with areas of signal void related to the presence of iron products.

■ Essential Facts

- Intramuscular myxoma is a solitary, benign soft-tissue tumor primarily affecting patients 40 to 70 years of age. It is more common in women.
- This paucicellular lesion contains abundant mucoid substance, which accounts for the T2 signal characteristics.
- The mass is most frequently located in the large muscles of the thigh, shoulder, or buttocks.
- Patients present with a firm, painless, palpable, and slowly enlarging soft-tissue mass.
- Treatment is local surgical excision. Recurrences are rare.

✔ Pearls & ✘ Pitfalls

- ✔ A peritumoral fat rind is visible on T1-weighted MR images, with increased signal intensity of the adjacent muscle on T2-weighted images.
- ✘ The tumors may have imaging features similar to those of myxoid liposarcoma.

Case 31

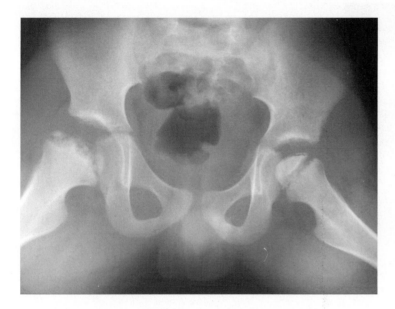

■ Clinical Presentation

The patient is an 8-year-old white male with bilateral hip pain.

■ Imaging Findings

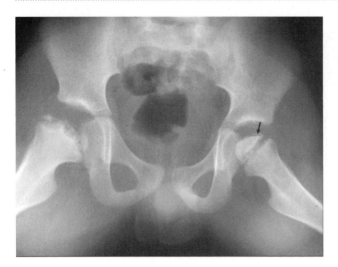

Imaging of both hips shows broadening of the right femoral neck and metaphysis with epiphyseal fragmentation and acetabular remodeling. The left hip demonstrates epiphyseal sclerosis and a "crescent sign" (*arrow*).

■ Differential Diagnosis

- **Legg-Calvé-Perthes disease:** A bilateral asymmetric pattern of osteonecrosis with fragmented/sclerotic epiphyses and a "crescent sign" are classic features of this diagnosis.
- *Hypothyroidism:* This is a symmetric process with characteristic laboratory abnormalities.
- *Sickle cell anemia:* This is a symmetric process that typically occurs in the black population.

■ Essential Facts

- Legg-Calvé-Perthes disease is an idiopathic form of avascular necrosis of the hips that is most likely related to vascular occlusion.
- The typical patient is a white male between 3 and 12 years of age.
- Bilateral asymmetric involvement is seen in ~15% of cases.
- Patients present with pain and limping.
- Treatment remains controversial. Some cases resolve, whereas others progress to osteoarthritis.
- Radiographs are the best screening tool.

✔ Pearls & ✗ Pitfalls

- ✔ The ossific nucleus of the femoral head may show subtle lateral displacement.
- ✗ It is not unusual to have normal findings on plain radiographs early in this disease process.

Case 32

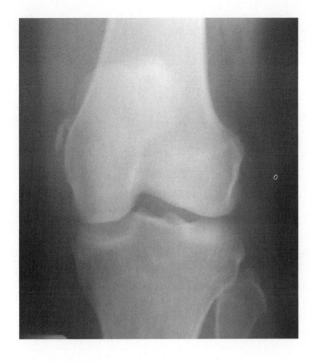

■ Clinical Presentation

The patient is a 40-year-old man with a history of chronic left knee pain and sprains.

■ Imaging Findings

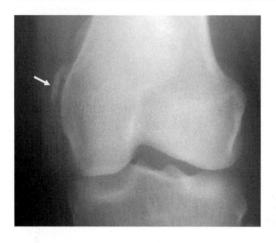

A frontal knee radiograph reveals smooth, curvilinear ossification along the periphery of the proximal medial femoral condyle (white arrow). No acute bony abnormality is evident.

■ Differential Diagnosis

- **Pellegrini-Stieda disease:** Localized smooth ossification along the medial femoral condyle in a patient with this history is characteristic of the diagnosis.
- *Crystalline deposition disease:* The fact that bone formation is seen excludes a crystalline deposition disease.
- *Avulsion fracture:* The rounded, smooth contour of the bone formation excludes an acute fracture/avulsion injury.

■ Essential Facts

- Pellegrini-Stieda disease reflects ossification of the medial collateral ligament (MCL) near the margin of the medial femoral condyle.
- Ossification is felt to be the result of healed past trauma to the MCL.

✔ Pearls & ✗ Pitfalls

- ✔ Curvilinear ossification adjacent to the femoral insertion of the MCL is diagnostic of Pellegrini-Stieda disease.
- ✗ Capsular heterotopic bone formation may mimic this process.

Case 33

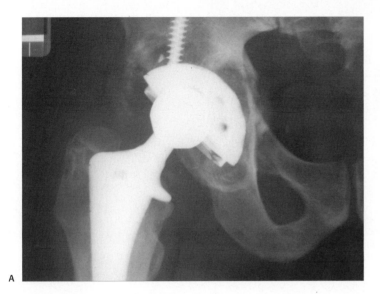

A

■ Clinical Presentation

The patient has a 6-month history of pain in the right hip.

Further Work-up

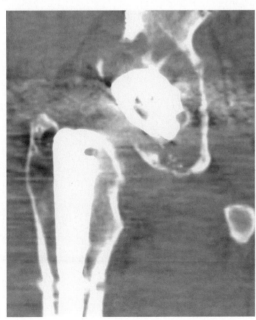

B

■ Imaging Findings

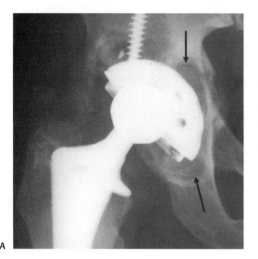
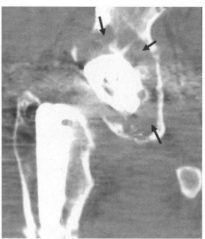

A   B

(A) Radiograph of the right hip shows total arthroplasty changes. Localized scalloped osteolytic regions (*black arrows*) enclose the acetabular cup. The femoral head shows superior eccentric positioning in the acetabulum. A healing fracture extends through the medial acetabular wall. **(B)** A coronal reformatted computed tomographic scan demonstrates soft-tissue density within the osteolytic regions along the acetabulum (*arrows*).

■ Differential Diagnosis

- ***Particle disease:*** The locally aggressive scalloped osteolysis in conjunction with an eccentrically positioned femoral head component and the absence of fever are consistent with particle disease.
- *Osteomyelitis:* The clinical presentation and pattern of nonconforming osteolysis with hardware malalignment are atypical of this process.

■ Essential Facts

- Particle disease is also known as aggressive granulomatosis.
- It is related to a histiocytic response of the bone to small polyethylene particles shed from the articular lining of orthopedic hardware.
- Localized osteolysis results after particles migrate and react with bone at the hardware interface.
- Abnormal liner wear may be evident by a superiorly malpositioned femoral head component.
- Patients may be asymptomatic until the bony changes are extensive enough to cause mechanical loosening of the hardware.
- This process is a relatively common reason for revision hip arthroplasty.

✔ Pearls & ✗ Pitfalls

- ✔ Particle disease may be distinguished from infection based on the absence of night pain and fever. Radiographic findings of nonconforming scalloped bone loss surrounding the hardware are typical. Regions of lucency > 2 mm surrounding the hardware should alert the radiologist to component loosening.
- ✗ Residual degenerative subcortical cystic changes in the native bone may mimic this disease process, emphasizing the utility of comparison films.

Case 34

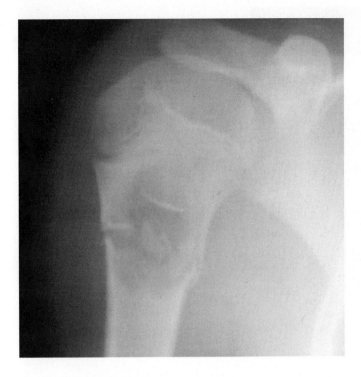

Clinical Presentation

The patient is a child who fell while playing at recess.

■ Imaging Findings

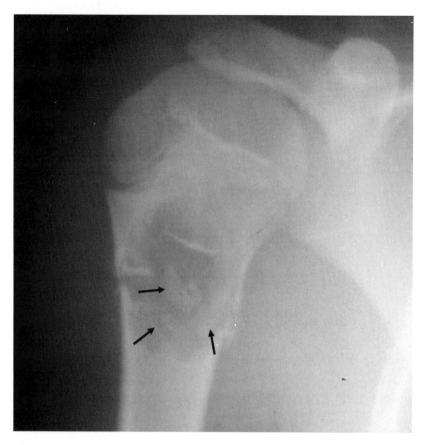

Radiograph of the shoulder displays a circumscribed osteolytic process centered in the proximal humerus, which demonstrates cortical thinning. A pathologic fracture is present. Multiple fragments positioned in the dependent region of the lesion (*arrows*) represent the "fallen fragment" sign.

■ Differential Diagnosis

- **Unicameral bone cyst:** A circumscribed lytic lesion in this location in a patient between 5 and 15 years of age is characteristic of the process.
- *Aneurysmal bone cyst:* The expansile nature of this lesion along with the soap bubble appearance are lacking in this case.
- *Fibrous dysplasia:* The absence of a "ground glass" appearance and the location are atypical of this monostotic lesion.

■ Essential Facts

- Unicameral bone cyst is a non-neoplastic, solitary, fluid-filled intraosseous cyst. It is also referred to as a simple bone cyst.
- It most commonly occurs in children between 5 and 15 years of age and is more frequent in boys.
- Characteristic locations include the proximal humerus and proximal femur.
- Patients commonly present with acute pain related to a fracture.

✔ Pearls & ✘ Pitfalls

- ✔ A "fallen fragment" sign is considered pathognomonic for this lesion.
- ✘ Septa may develop in the lesion, complicating the diagnosis.

Case 35

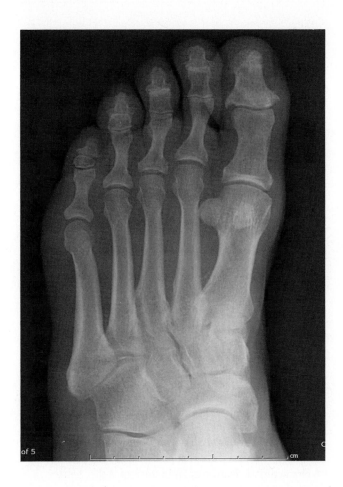

Clinical Presentation

A 64-year-old man presents with polyarthralgias and foot pain.

■ Imaging Findings

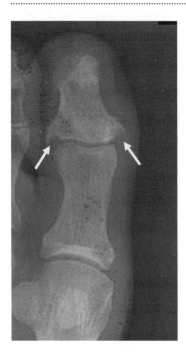

Radiograph of the foot shows marginal erosions of bone with adjacent, irregular proliferation of bone in the interphalangeal joint of the great toe (*arrows*). Slightly increased density of the distal phalanx is seen.

■ Differential Diagnosis

- ***Psoriatic arthritis (PA):*** Involvement of the interphalangeal joint of the great toe with an admixture of periarticular erosions and proliferation of bone in an asymmetric distribution in a patient with polyarthralgias raises suspicion for PA. Increased density of the distal phalanx ("ivory phalanx") further supports this diagnosis.
- *Gout:* The proliferation of bone and para-articular erosions at the first metatarsal-phalangeal joint are lacking.
- *Reactive arthritis:* Supporting signs and symptoms of prior genitourinary tract infection are lacking, and this patient is older than is usual for reactive arthritis.

■ Essential Facts

- PA is a chronic, inflammatory, proliferative disease of the skin.
- It commonly affects whites.
- Genetic, environmental, and immunologic factors have been considered to have key roles in the development and expression of PA.
- As many as 60% of patients are seropositive for HLA-B27.
- The mean age at diagnosis of PA is 40 years.
- Skin manifestations precede the development of arthritis, which may be bilateral or unilateral and symmetric or asymmetric.
- The hands and feet are the most commonly involved locations in PA.
- The involvement of several joints in a single digit, with soft-tissue swelling, produces what appears clinically as a "sausage digit."

- Erosion of bone typically begins at the margins of the joint and continues along the articular surface or progresses along the joint capsule away from the joint.
- Proliferation of bone produces an irregular and indistinct appearance of the marginal bone about the involved joint, characterized as a "fuzzy" appearance or "whiskering."
- A characteristic feature of PA in the foot is the "ivory phalanx," which classically involves the distal phalanges (especially in the first digit) and is comprised of sclerosis, enthesitis, periostitis, and soft-tissue swelling.
- Bone mineralization is typically preserved.

✔ Pearls & ✗ Pitfalls

- ✔ Proliferation of bone is especially prominent in PA and is the most distinguishing feature of this condition. Distal interphalangeal joint involvement is usually present in the hands and feet.
- ✗ Given the asymmetric monoarticular distribution, PA may mimic an infectious process.

Case 36

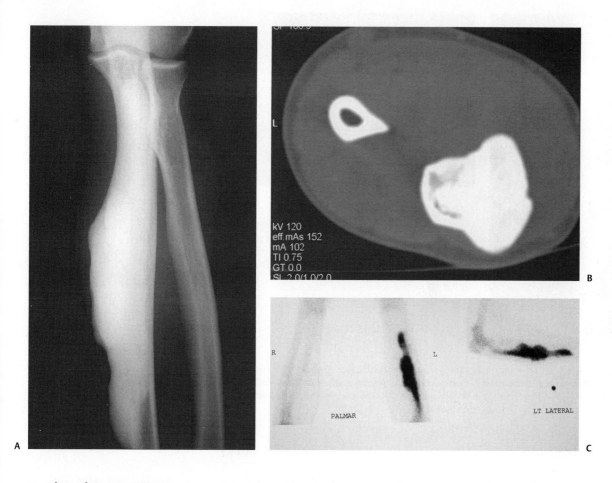

■ Clinical Presentation

A 25-year-old man presents with a palpable bony mass and stiffness in the left forearm.

■ Imaging Findings

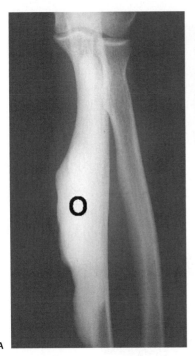
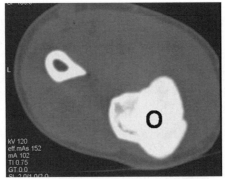
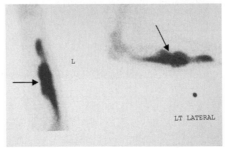

(A) Radiograph of the left forearm shows dense, flowing, segmental ossification (*O*) along the ulnar diaphysis. **(B)** Axial computed tomographic scan shows dense, organized ossification (*O*) applied to the medial ulnar cortex with medullary involvement and no soft-tissue abnormality. **(C)** Nuclear medicine bone scan of the forearm illustrates avid uptake (*arrows*).

■ Differential Diagnosis

- **Melorheostosis:** Dense, flowing, segmental ossification extending along the unicortical length of a long bone is characteristic.
- *Paget's disease:* This disease is seen in older patients and expands and coarsens the trabecular bone.
- *Osteosarcoma:* The organized, dense bone formation without a soft-tissue component or periosteal reaction is not typical of this malignancy.

■ Essential Facts

- Melorheostosis is a bone-forming dystrophy leading to irregular thickening of cortical bone.
- This is felt to be a developmental error primarily in intramembranous bone formation with overproduction of bone matrix in skeletal regions innervated by a single spinal sensory nerve.
- Patients manifest clinically with limb stiffness or pain.
- The disease usually remains occult until late adolescence or early adulthood.
- It follows a chronic, progressive course, occasionally resulting in substantial disability that may lead to amputation.
- It is common in the long bones of the upper and lower extremities.

✔ Pearls & ✗ Pitfalls

- ✔ Melorheostosis typically involves one side of the cortical bone and extends to but does not pass the articular surface.
- ✗ Melorheostosis may coexist with the other bone-forming dystrophies: osteopoikilosis and osteopathia striata.

Case 37

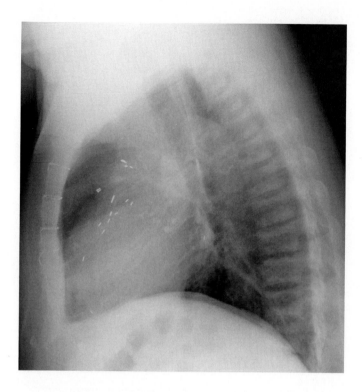

■ **Clinical Presentation**

The patient has undergone a preoperative work-up for a kidney transplant.

■ Imaging Findings

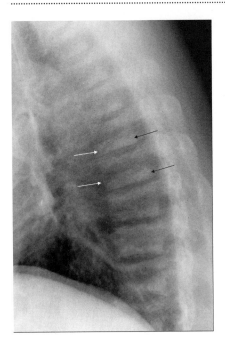

A lateral radiograph of the chest reveals bandlike areas of sclerosis adjacent to the vertebral body end plates (*arrows*), an appearance that has been likened to the stripes on rugby jerseys ("rugger jersey spine").

■ Differential Diagnosis

- **Rugger jersey spine:** Thick bands of sclerosis at the end plates of multiple vertebral bodies in a patient with renal disease is characteristic of rugger jersey spine related to secondary hyperparathyroidism.
- *Paget's disease:* This disease typically affects a single vertebral body and causes focal enlargement of the vertebral body.
- *Osteoporosis:* The bandlike densities are too thick for this diagnosis; additionally, no fragility fractures or "fish vertebrae" are seen.

■ Essential Facts

- Rugger jersey spine describes the striped sclerotic changes affecting the vertebrae in secondary hyperparathyroidism.
- The opaque sclerotic bands seen on the inferior and superior end plates of vertebral bodies represent excess accumulations of osteoid related to osteoblastic activity resulting from abnormally high levels of parathyroid hormone.
- Osteosclerosis due to renal osteodystrophy tends to predominate in the axial skeleton, most commonly manifesting in the pelvis, ribs, and spine.

✔ Pearls & ✘ Pitfalls

- ✔ Rugger jersey spine is a multisegmental process affecting multiple vertebral bodies and is not uncommonly diagnosed on lateral chest radiographs.
- ✘ Sclerotic vertebral body metastases may occasionally resemble "rugger jersey spine."

Case 38

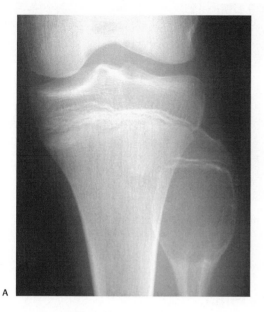

A

■ Clinical Presentation

A 17-year-old patient presents with pain in the left leg.

Further Work-up

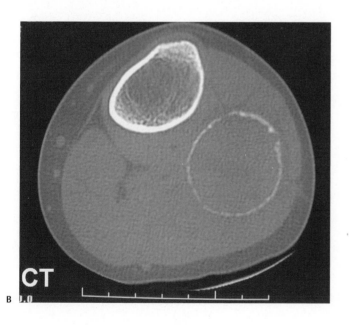

B

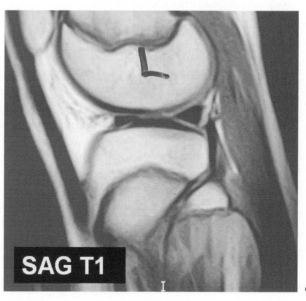

C

■ Imaging Findings

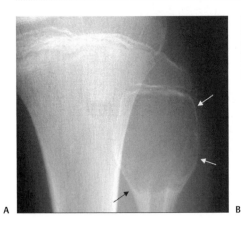

A

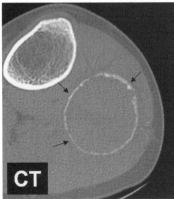

B

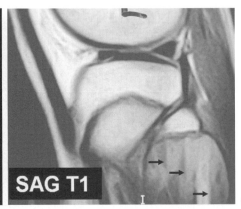

C

(A) Radiograph of the proximal portion of the tibia and fibula shows a circumscribed expansile, lytic lesion in the proximal fibular metaphysis (*arrows*). Both cortices are ballooned. There is no soft-tissue mass or internal mineralization. **(B,C)** Axial computed tomographic scan shows thinned cortices (*arrows*) with no matrix mineralization. Sagittal T1-weighted magnetic resonance imaging (MRI) demonstrates fluid-fluid levels (*arrows*) with no solid component.

■ Differential Diagnosis

- *Aneurysmal bone cyst (ABC):* A localized expansile, lytic lesion in a long bone with marked cortical thinning exhibiting fluid-fluid levels on MRI is classic for ABC.
- *Fibrous dysplasia:* The absence of a "ground glass" matrix and the localized expansile nature of this process argue against fibrous dysplasia.
- *Simple bone cyst:* The location and expansile nature of this lesion are atypical of a simple bone cyst.

■ Essential Facts

- ABC is a benign lesion of bone related to a reactive vascular process.
- The vascular process is responsible for the fluid-fluid levels evident on MRI and the expansile aneurysmal appearance on plain film.
- ABCs may represent a secondary hemorrhagic process related to an antecedent solid tumor, such as giant cell tumor, chondroblastoma, or fibrous dysplasia.
- More than 80% of primary ABCs occur in patients younger than 20 years of age, who present with localized pain and swelling.
- The lesion predominates in the metaphyseal regions of long bones.
- Treatment is with curettage.

✔ Pearls & ✗ Pitfalls

- ✔ Spinal ABCs tend to involve the posterior elements.
- ✗ This lesion may occasionally demonstrate periostitis with a Codman triangle.

Case 39

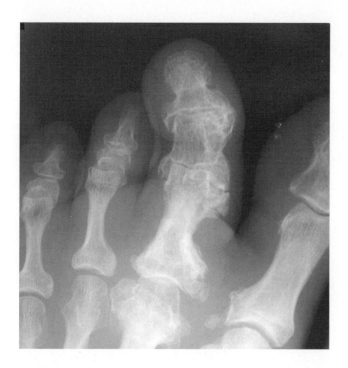

■ Clinical Presentation
....

A 25-year-old man presents with a deformed foot.

■ Imaging Findings

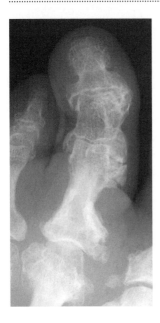

Radiographic view of the phalanges of the foot shows overgrowth of the bony structures of the second digit with lateral osseous bowing. Osteoarthritic changes are seen extending proximally into the metatarsophalangeal joint.

■ Differential Diagnosis

- *Macrodystrophia lipomatosa:* Enlargement of a single digit unilaterally in a lower extremity with involvement of the second or third phalanx is characteristic of this diagnosis.
- *Neurofibromatosis type 1:* This process may cause digital enlargement bilaterally.
- *Klippel-Trénaunay-Weber syndrome:* Cutaneous abnormalities are typically present.

■ Essential Facts

- Macrodystrophia lipomatosa is also known as localized gigantism or macrodactyly. It presents before the age of 30 years, most commonly at birth or in early childhood.
- Enlargement of a single digit is seen unilaterally. If two digits are involved, they are adjacent.
- There is no known cause or hereditary predisposition. The upper extremity is affected more frequently than the lower extremity.
- A fibrolipomatous hamartoma involves the nerve innervating the affected phalanx.
- Macrodactyly results in disproportionate overgrowth of surrounding fibroadipose tissue.
- The digit often displays osteoarthritic change.
- It may be treated with amputation because of the extensive associated deformity.
- Digit growth ceases at puberty.

✔ Pearls & ✗ Pitfalls

- ✔ Overgrowth of bone is typically more prominent distally and on the volar side of the digit. This lesion tends to involve the second and third rays of the hand or foot.
- ✗ The bony overgrowth may not be as obvious as the soft-tissue/fatty hypertrophy, making radiographic detection difficult.

Case 40

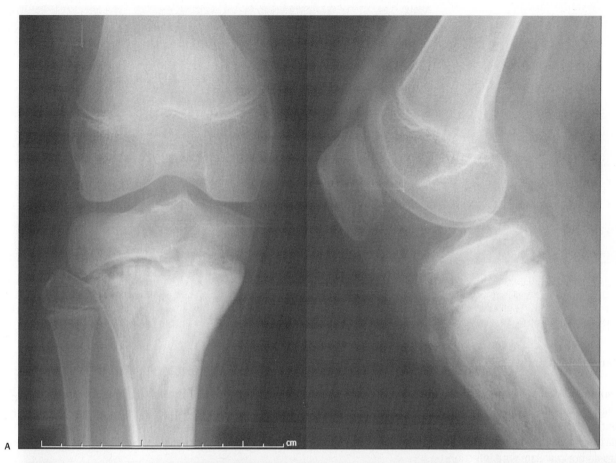

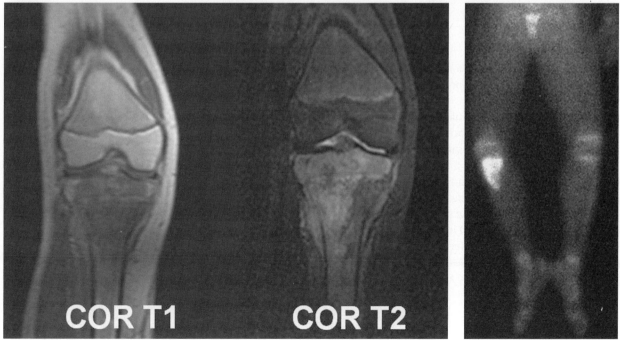

Clinical Presentation

A 13-year-old patient presents with a 6-month history of knee pain.

■ Imaging Findings

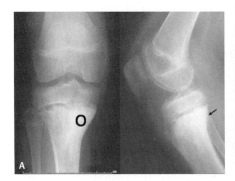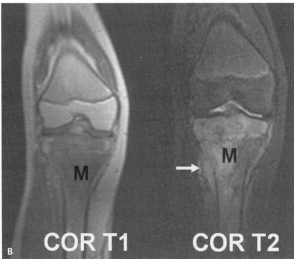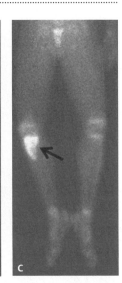

(A) Radiographs of the knee show a tibial metaphyseal medulla-based osteoblastic process (*O*) with periosteal reaction (*arrows*). **(B)** Magnetic resonance imaging (MRI) shows an intramedullary mass (*M*) in the tibial metaphysis with extension into the epiphysis, not seen on radiographs. The lesion shows low signal intensity on T1- and T2-weighted images. A soft-tissue component (*arrows*) is evident. **(C)** A bone scan shows isotope uptake in the tibia (*arrow*), correlating with the MRI findings.

■ Differential Diagnosis

- *Osteosarcoma:* A tibial metaphyseal medullary-based osteoblastic mass with periostitis and a soft-tissue component in this age group is classic for osteosarcoma.
- *Chronic osteomyelitis:* The patient's presentation and MRI findings do not correlate with infection.

■ Essential Facts

- Osteosarcoma, a malignant bone-forming tumor, is the most common primary bone tumor of adolescents and young adults.
- Numerous variants of osteosarcoma exist and can involve the medullary canal, cortical surface, or soft tissues.
- The intramedullary form of osteosarcoma is the most common.
- Patients may present with pain and swelling, typically in the second and third decades of life.
- MRI is ideal for assessing bony and soft-tissue involvement, with bone scanning used to identify metastasis.
- Osteosarcoma most frequently affects the long bones about the knee.
- Treatment includes chemotherapy and surgery.

✔ Pearls & ✘ Pitfalls

- ✔ Pulmonary metastasis from osteosarcoma can manifest as a spontaneous pneumothorax.
- ✘ The radiographic diagnosis of lytic osteosarcomas can be challenging, given the decreased osteoid formation.

Case 41

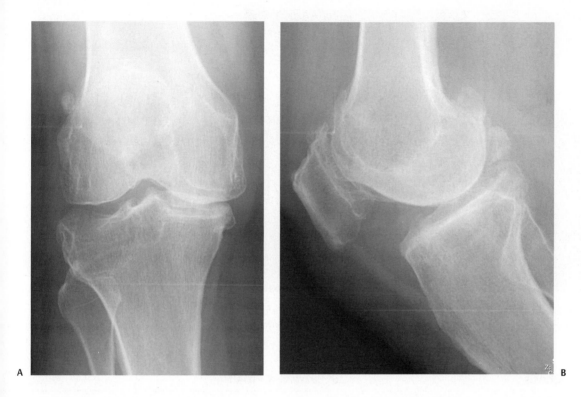

A

B

◼ Clinical Presentation

A 57-year-old woman presents with chronic knee pain.

■ Imaging Findings

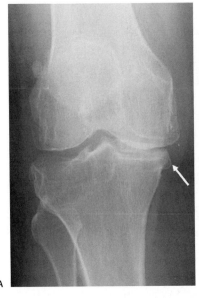 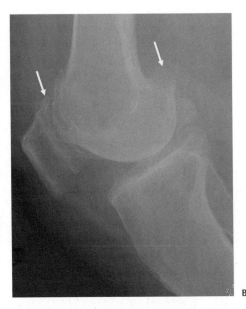

A   B

(A,B) Radiographs of the knee show joint space narrowing, sclerosis, and extensive osteophyte formation (*arrows*) predominantly involving the medial femorotibial and patellofemoral compartments. No osteopenia is present.

■ Differential Diagnosis

- **Osteoarthrosis:** The pattern of joint space narrowing with sclerosis and osteophyte formation is typical of osteoarthrosis.
- *Neuropathic joint:* Destructive bony fragmentation, articular collapse, and subluxation are absent in this patient.
- *Calcium phosphate dihydrate (CPPD) arthropathy:* The absence of chondrocalcinosis, extensive subcortical cystic change, and disproportionate patellofemoral arthropathy dismisses this diagnosis.

■ Essential Facts

- Osteoarthrosis results from articular cartilage damage caused by repetitive microtrauma that occurs throughout life.
- It tends to involve specific synovial joints during specific decades of a person's life and depends in part on the patient's body habitus and level of physical activity.
- In the knee joints, joint space narrowing is typically asymmetric and most commonly involves the medial femorotibial compartment and possibly the patellofemoral compartment.
- The presence of osteophytes, bone sclerosis, and subchondral cysts and the absence of inflammatory features such as erosions suggest this diagnosis.
- As the joint space narrows, the osteophytes become larger, bone sclerosis increases, and the formation of subchondral cysts, or geodes, may be seen.

✔ Pearls & ✘ Pitfalls

- ✔ A weight-bearing radiograph will improve the detection of early joint space narrowing.
- ✘ Several causes of secondary cartilage damage may be associated with atypical osteoarthrosis.

Case 42

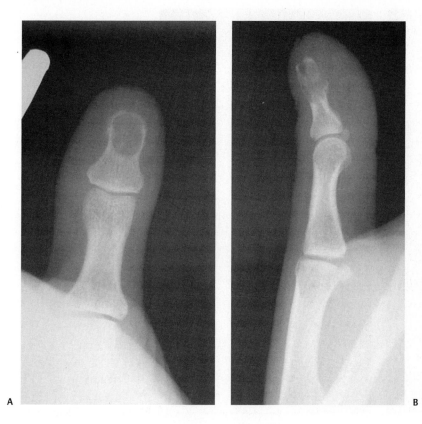

A

B

■ Clinical Presentation

A 40-year-old man who has a remote history of penetrating injury to the thumb presents with swelling.

■ Imaging Findings

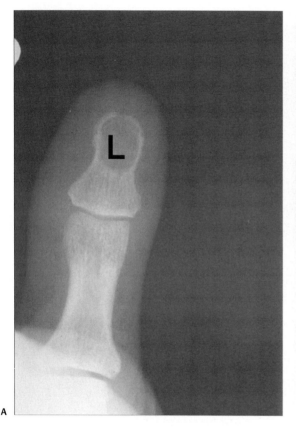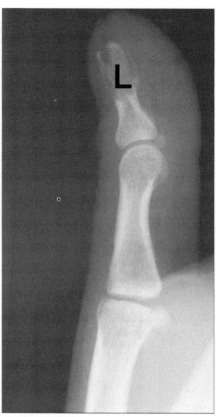

A   B

(A,B) Radiographs of the thumb show a well-defined, nonmineralized, unilocular, osteolytic lesion (*L*) of the terminal phalanx with mild soft-tissue swelling.

■ Differential Diagnosis

- *Epidermal inclusion cyst (EIC):* The location within the terminal phalanx, circumscribed lytic bony changes, and clinical history are distinct features of an EIC.
- *Glomus tumor:* This lesion tends to cause extrinsic erosion along the terminal phalanx subjacent to the nail bed and is extremely tender to palpation.
- *Enchondroma:* This tumor is rare in the thumb and terminal phalanges.

■ Essential Facts

- EIC is a benign, nonaggressive tumor.
- It is thought to be related to penetrating trauma, which allows the intraosseous deposition of epidermal cells that proliferate.
- Central keratinized debris develops within the lytic lesion and is seen on radiographs.
- EIC is three times more common in men and occurs in persons between 25 and 50 years of age.
- The sites most commonly affected with this lesion are the terminal phalanges of the hand.
- Patients can present with pain, swelling, and tenderness. Local excision is curative.

✔ Pearls & ✘ Pitfalls

- ✔ The most common site of localized involvement with an EIC is the terminal phalanx of the middle finger.
- ✘ Pathologic evaluation of the lesion is typically required for a definitive diagnosis.

Case 43

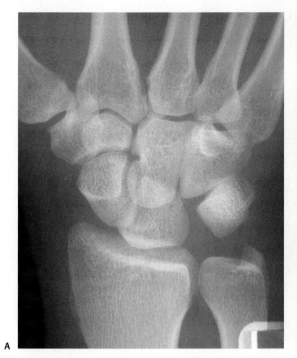

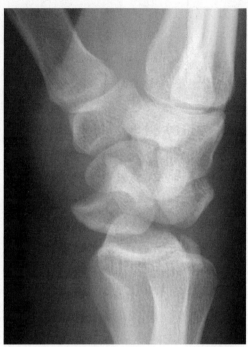

A   B

■ Clinical Presentation

The patient has fallen onto an outstretched hand.

■ Imaging Findings

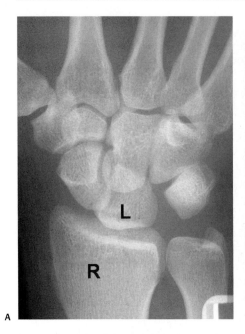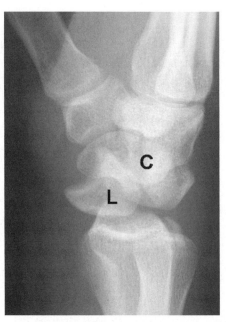

A   B

(A,B) Radiographs of the wrist demonstrate volar rotation of the lunate (*L*) with disruption of the articulations with the capitate (*C*) and radius (*R*). The lunate has a characteristic triangular shape on the frontal view related to the rotational changes.

■ Differential Diagnosis

- **Lunate dislocation:** Ventral disarticulation/rotation of the lunate from the capitate and radial articular surfaces is classic for this injury.

■ Essential Facts

- Ventral lunate dislocation is the fourth stage of progressive perilunate instability.
- The first three stages are scapholunate dissociation, perilunate dislocation, and disruption of the radiotriquetral/lunotriquetral ligament.
- This is a hyperextension injury in which the capitate forces the lunate ventrally.
- It commonly occurs secondary to a fall onto an outstretched hand.

✔ Pearls & ✗ Pitfalls

- ✔ This entity can be associated with a dorsal radiolunate ligament injury.
- ✗ The lunate and capitate can falsely appear aligned with the radial articular surface on poorly positioned lateral views.

Case 44

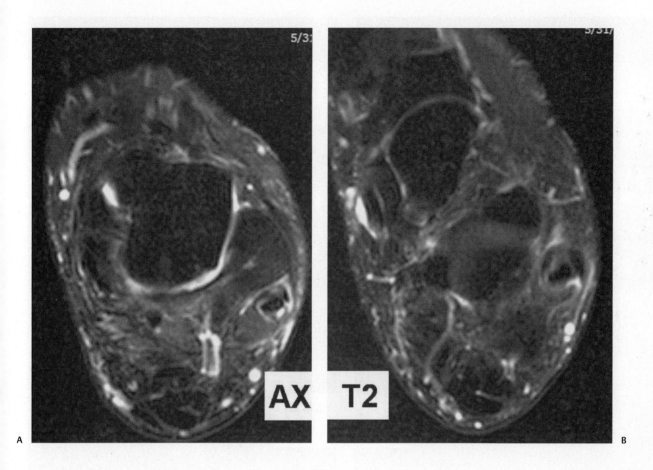

A   AX   T2   B

■ **Clinical Presentation**

The patient is a 36-year-old man with chronic lateral ankle pain.

■ Imaging Findings

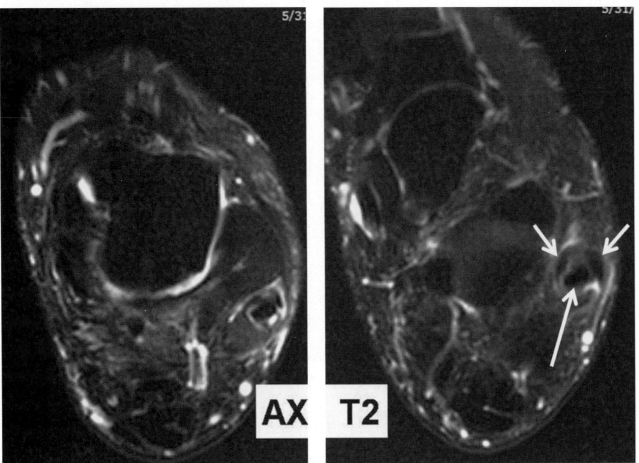

A　　　　　　　　　　　　　　　　　　　　　　　　　　　　　　　　　　　B

(A,B) Axial T2-weighted magnetic resonance imaging (MRI) demonstrates a C-shaped split peroneus brevis tendon (*short white arrows*) partially enveloping the peroneus longus tendon (*long white arrow*).

■ Differential Diagnosis

- ***Split peroneus brevis tendon:*** Longitudinal intrasubstance interruption, or a C-shaped or "boomerang" configuration of this tendon that partially envelops the peroneus longus tendon, represents this type of tear.

■ Essential Facts

- Split peroneus brevis tendon is related to overuse in young athletes or degenerative wear and tear in older, more sedentary patients.
- Longitudinal split tears often originate within the fibular groove, where the tendon is entrapped between the peroneus longus tendon and the lateral malleolus.
- Partial or full substance splits within the tendon show intrasubstance high signal intensity on axial T2-weighted MRI.
- They may be associated with superior peroneal retinacular tears or be secondary to inversion ankle injuries.
- Calcaneal fractures can predispose to partial tears, dislocation, and entrapment.

✔ Pearls & ✘ Pitfalls

- ✔ Tears commonly occur at the lateral malleolus secondary to the frictional 90-degree turn. The C-shape of a normal peroneus brevis tendon should never be thinner centrally than peripherally.
- ✘ A normal peroneus brevis tendon often assumes a C-shape at the lateral malleolus.

Case 45

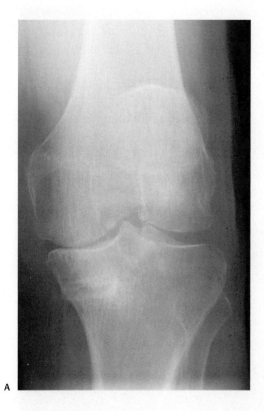

A

■ Clinical Presentation

A 74-year-old woman presents with chronic knee pain and no history of trauma.

Further Work-up

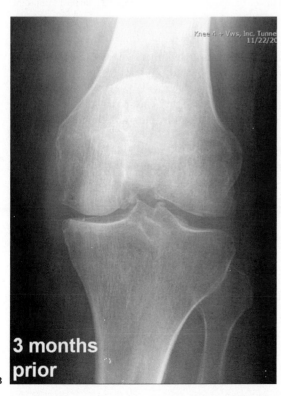

3 months prior

B

■ Imaging Findings

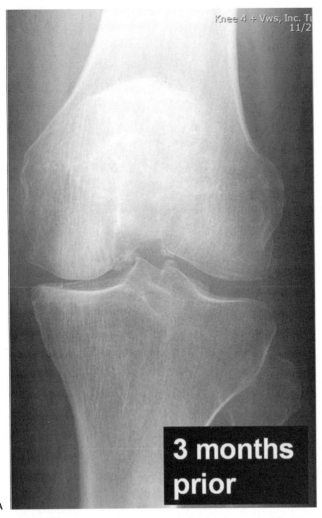
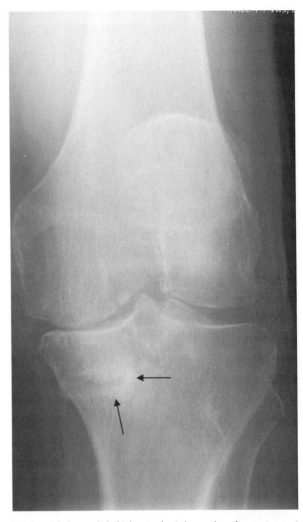

A   B

Radiographs of the knee show a bandlike area of lucency enclosed by sclerosis extending through the medial tibial metaphysis (*arrows*) on the most recent film (**B**). This was not demonstrated on a radiograph performed 3 months earlier (**A**). Mild osteopenia is evident.

■ Differential Diagnosis

• **Insufficiency fracture:** A lucent defect surrounded by sclerosis in the medial tibial metaphysis of an elderly woman with osteopenia is characteristic of an insufficiency fracture.

■ Essential Facts

• Insufficiency fractures result from the application of normal physiologic forces to weakened bone, most often osteoporotic bone, as in this case.
• Other causes besides osteoporosis include Paget's disease, rheumatoid arthritis, and metabolic bone diseases.
• The area of lucency on radiographs represents the fracture defect; surrounding sclerosis is related to remodeling.

• The typical patient is an elderly woman with osteopenia and no prior history of trauma who presents with localized pain.
• Typical locations include the pubic rami, sacrum, and lower extremities. Early on, radiograph findings are normal.
• Early detection is possible with magnetic resonance imaging and bone scan, which show areas of abnormal signal on T1- and T2-weighted images and increased uptake of radiotracer, respectively.

✔ Pearls & ✗ Pitfalls

✔ Comparison films, if available, can commonly assist with the diagnosis.
✗ Radiographic findings may be negative for several weeks.

Case 46

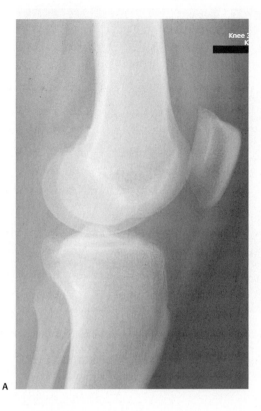

A

■ Clinical Presentation

The patient is a 19-year-old man who sustained a twisting injury while playing soccer.

Further Work-up

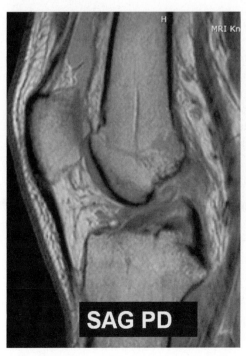

B

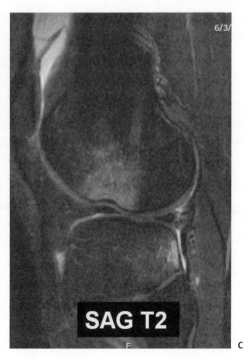

C

■ Imaging Findings

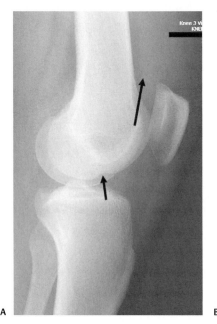
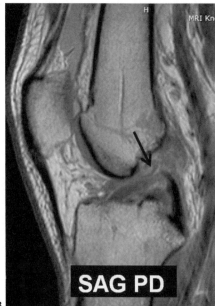
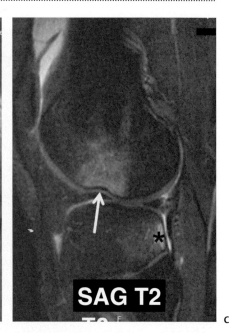

A   B   C

(A) Radiograph of the knee show an abnormally deep depression over the lateral condylopatellar sulcus (*short arrow*). A large joint effusion (*long arrow*) is also present. **(B,C)** Sagittal proton density (PD)-weighted and T2-weighted magnetic resonance imaging (MRI) shows complete disruption of the anterior cruciate ligament (ACL: *black arrow*). A depressed bone contu-sion is located anteriorly (*white arrow*) along the lateral femoral condyle, accounting for the deepening of the lateral femoral sulcus noted on the radiographs. A kissing contusion involves the posterior lateral tibial plateau (*asterisk*).

■ Differential Diagnosis

• **Anterior cruciate ligament tear:** A deepened lateral condylopatellar sulcus (lateral femoral notch sign) with a joint effusion and a history of a twisting injury are indirect signs and symptoms of a torn ACL. The lateral femoral notch sign/contusion and posterior fracture/contusion of the lateral tibial plateau seen on MRI represent kissing contusions. The disrupted fibers of the ACL confirm the diagnosis.

■ Essential Facts

• ACL injuries occur when a valgus load is applied to the knee in various states of flexion combined with external rotation of the tibia or internal rotation of the femur.
• This type of injury usually occurs during maneuvers such as rapid deceleration and simultaneous change of direction.
• These maneuvers load the ACL and can cause it to rupture.
• Once the ACL is disrupted, anterior subluxation of the tibia relative to the femur occurs, which results in impaction of the lateral femoral condyle against the posterolateral margin of the lateral tibial plateau.

• Disruption most commonly occurs in the midsubstance of the ACL. Other soft-tissue injuries include tears of the posterior capsule and arcuate ligament, the posterior horn of the lateral or medial meniscus, and the medial collateral ligament.
• Surgical repair is required.

✔ Pearls & ✘ Pitfalls

✔ A depression in the lateral femoral condyle > 2.0 mm deep is highly suggestive of an ACL injury
✘ Difficulty may arise in distinguishing between a prominent but normal lateral condylopatellar sulcus and a shallow impacted fracture at the sulcus. The lateral femoral notch sign is not frequently encountered with ACL tears.

Case 47

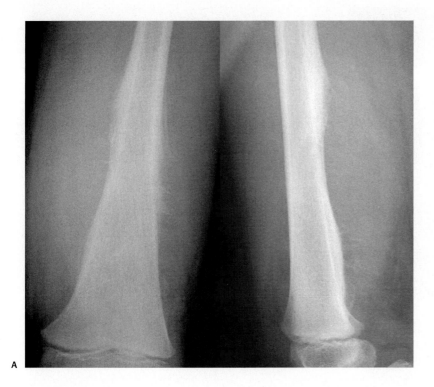

A

■ Clinical Presentation

The patient is a 15-year-old girl with pain and swelling of the left thigh for 4 months.

Further Work-up

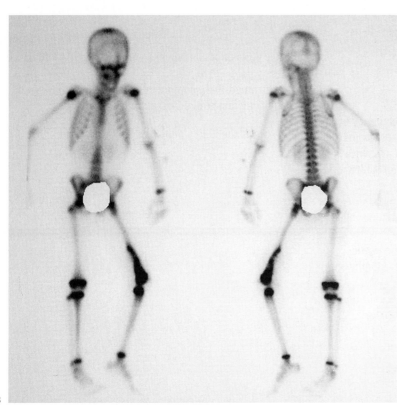

B

■ Imaging Findings

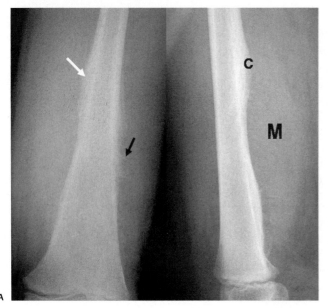

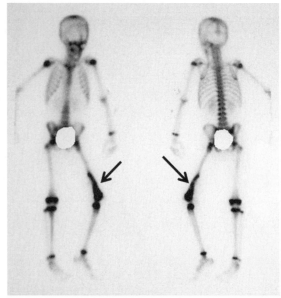

(A) Radiograph of the left femur display an aggressive-appearing segment of a lamellar (*white arrow*) and spiculated (*black arrow*) periosteal reaction with a Codman triangle (*c*) along the distal femoral diametaphysis. An associated soft-tissue mass (*M*) is present, causing a concave deformity over the external cortex of the femur. No matrix calcifications are seen. **(B)** Radionuclide bone scan shows increased activity (*arrows*) involving the distal half of the femur.

■ Differential Diagnosis

- **Ewing sarcoma:** An aggressive bony process containing a large soft-tissue component in the diametaphysis of a bone in the lower extremity of a young patient is highly suggestive of this sarcoma.
- *Osteosarcoma:* The absence of mineralized matrix formation makes osteosarcoma a less likely diagnosis.
- *Osteomyelitis:* The clinical presentation and large soft-tissue mass make infection unlikely.

■ Essential Facts

- Ewing sarcoma is the second most common malignancy of bone in children and adolescents, following osteosarcoma.
- The peak incidence is between 10 to 15 years of age, with a slight male predominance and a predilection for white individuals.
- Patients present with nonspecific pain or swelling.
- This tumor is a poorly differentiated small round blue cell tumor.
- It exhibits a predilection for the long bones of the lower extremity with localization to the diaphysis/metadiaphysis, where lytic/permeative bony changes can be seen.
- An associated nonmineralized soft-tissue mass is common and is caused by tumor extension through the cortical bone.

- The soft-tissue mass may encircle the affected bone, causing a saucerlike formation or concave mass effect on the underlying cortex.
- Bone scanning and magnetic resonance imaging are useful for evaluating the extent of disease.
- Treatment is with chemotherapy and resection.

✔ Pearls & ✗ Pitfalls

- ✔ Eighty percent of all Ewing sarcomas contain a soft-tissue mass.
- ✗ The intramedullary component of the tumor may not be easily detectable on radiographs.

Case 48

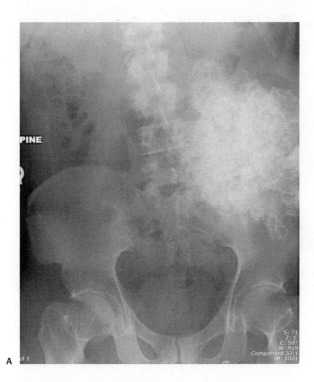

Clinical Presentation

A 34-year-old man presents with a 1-year history of an abdominal mass and weakness in the left lower extremity.

Further Work-up

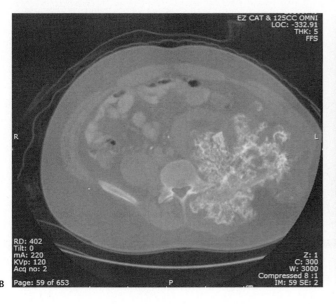

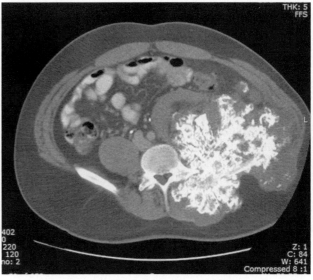

■ Imaging Findings

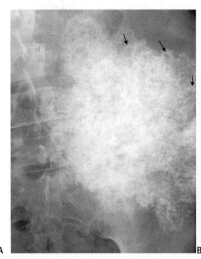
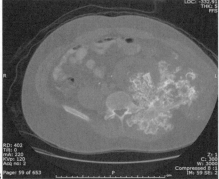
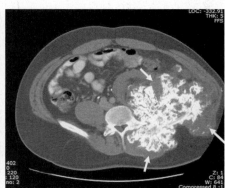

A B C

(A) Abdominal radiograph displays a large, densely mineralized mass occupying most of the left hemiabdomen. The calcifications have a chondroid appearance with a ringlike and arclike configuration (*arrows*). **(B,C)** Computed tomography scans show the chondroid calcifications to better advantage. The lesion replaces the left ilium and is encircled by a soft-tissue mass (*arrows*). The left-sided retroperitoneal structures are displaced medially.

■ Differential Diagnosis

- *Chondrosarcoma:* The lesion size of > 7 cm, chondroid calcifications, a soft-tissue mass, bony replacement, and history of pain are distinct for a chondrosarcoma.
- *Osteosarcoma:* The chondroid mineralization with a surrounding soft-tissue mass is not typical for osteosarcoma.
- *Osteochondroma:* The haphazard mineralization and aggressive growth do not favor osteochondroma.

■ Essential Facts

- Chondrosarcoma is the second most commonly encountered primary neoplasm of bone in adults.
- It typically presents insidiously with progressive pain.
- Patients present in the fourth to fifth decades; common sites include the pelvis and femur.
- This very cellular lesion is composed of atypical chondrocytes/multinucleated cells and exhibits an aggressive growth pattern that produces a large focus of marrow replacement with cortical destruction and a soft-tissue mass.
- Characteristic or atypical chondroid calcifications may be present depending on the degree of differentiation.
- Therapy is surgical excision.

✔ Pearls & ✘ Pitfalls

- ✔ Chondrosarcoma is rare in the feet and hands. Pain is a helpful clinical determinant.
- ✘ Sampling error during biopsy may lead to a false-negative diagnosis.

Case 49

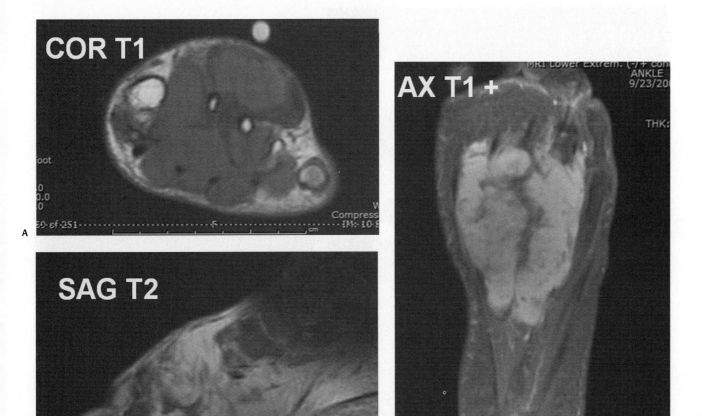

COR T1

SAG T2

AX T1 +

A

B

C

▦ Clinical Presentation

A 28-year-old woman presents with a 2-year history of an enlarging foot mass.

■ Imaging Findings

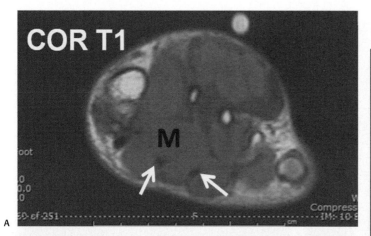

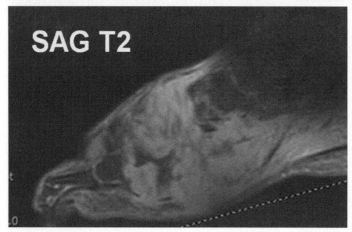

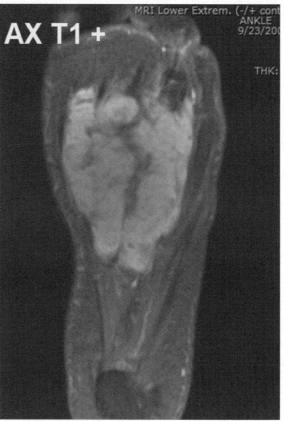

(A–C) Magnetic resonance imaging of the foot shows a solid lobulated mass (*M*) investing the plantar flexor tendons (*arrows*) extending into the dorsal soft tissues. The mass demonstrates isointense T1 and T2 signal relative to muscle with diffuse enhancement. No calcification or blooming artifact is evident.

■ Differential Diagnosis

- **Fibroma of the tendon sheath:** The lobulated morphology, low MR signal intensity, and encasement of the flexor tendons of the foot are distinct features of this diagnosis.
- *Giant cell tumor of the tendon sheath:* This tumor typically shows a lower signal intensity on T2-weighted imaging with blooming artifact.
- *Synovial sarcoma:* The absence of calcifications, osseous invasion, and a hyperintense signal on T2-weighted images exclude this entity.

■ Essential Facts

- Fibroma of the tendon sheath is a benign overgrowth of tissue containing a large quantity of collagen, which accounts for the low signal intensity on T1- and T2-weighted MR images.
- The upper extremities, particularly the fingers, hands, and wrists, are the site of the majority of lesions.

- Patients present with a slowly growing, painless soft-tissue mass, typically between the ages of 20 and 50 years.
- Men are affected twice as often as women.
- Local excision is the treatment of choice, with a recurrence rate as high as 24%.
- Fibroma of the tendon sheath and giant cell tumor of the tendon sheath may represent the two end points of a spectrum of cellular proliferation.

✔ Pearls & ✘ Pitfalls

- ✔ The hemosiderin deposition seen with giant cell tumor of the tendon sheath may cause blooming artifact, a feature that is not expected in a fibroma of the tendon sheath.
- ✘ Fibromas and giant cell tumors of the tendon sheath occur in a similar patient population, and both present as painless, slowly growing masses.

Case 50

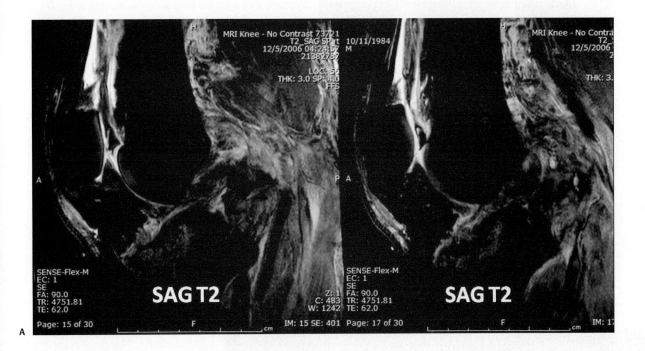

Clinical Presentation

A 22-year-old man has sustained severe trauma to the knee.

Further Work-up

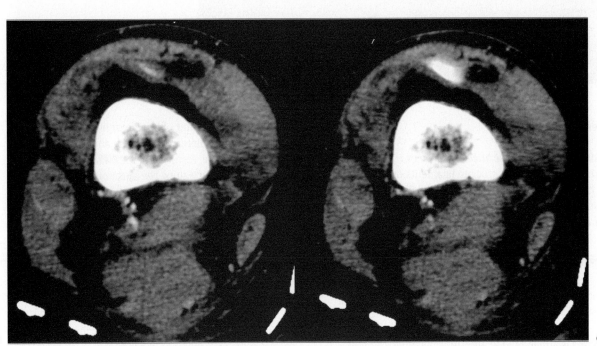

■ Imaging Findings

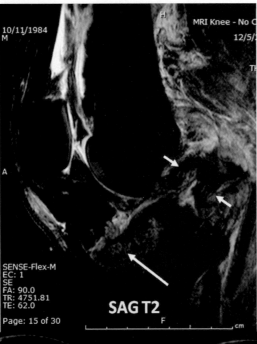

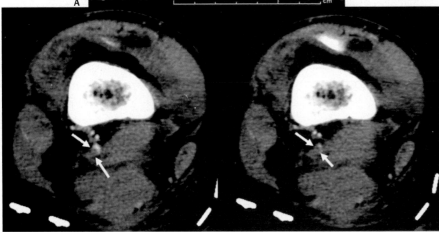

(A) Sagittal T2-weighted magnetic resonance (MR) image of the knee shows absence of the cruciate ligaments with replacement by disorganized fibers (*short arrows*). Edema is superimposed on a fracture over the anterior margin of the tibia (*long arrow*). **(B,C)** Axial computed tomographic angiogram shows an irregular filling defect (*arrows*) in the popliteal artery, indicating a traumatic thrombus.

■ Differential Diagnosis

• **Anterior dislocation of the knee:** Absence or rupture of the anterior and posterior cruciate ligaments on MR images is most consistent with femoral-tibial dislocation. The anterior proximal tibial fracture represents an anterior dislocation mechanism.

■ Essential Facts

• Anterior dislocation of the knee, the most common type, is typically seen following a forceful blow to an extended knee.
• Direct force is applied to the anterior tibia while the foot is planted, or the dislocation may result from an indirect force, such as a forceful kicking motion.
• Severe cases often result from direct injury, as when the bumper of a car hits the anterior tibia of a pedestrian.

• During the brief moment of hyperextension, the anterior aspect of the tibial plateau strikes the anterior aspect of the femoral condyle, resulting in the "kissing" contusion pattern of bone injury along the anterior tibia and femur.
• The posterior cruciate ligament ruptures initially, and if the force continues, the anterior cruciate ligament fails.
• Injury of the popliteal artery is seen in up to 50% of cases.
• Disruption of the posterolateral complex and possibly gastrocnemius injury can occur.

✔ Pearls & ✗ Pitfalls

✔ Evaluation of the popliteal neurovascular bundle is mandatory in the management of combined acute anterior and posterior cruciate ligament injuries.
✗ Not all dislocations of the knee involve combined tearing of the anterior and posterior cruciate ligaments.

Case 51

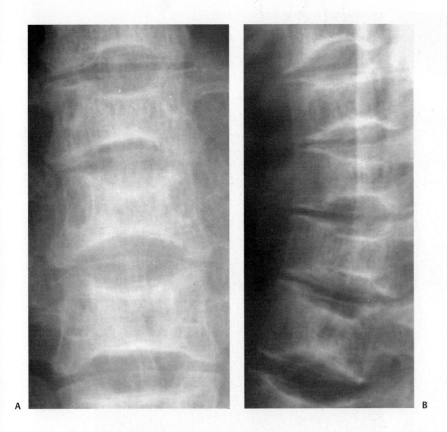

A   B

▨ Clinical Presentation

A 26-year-old black man presents with back pain.

■ Imaging Findings

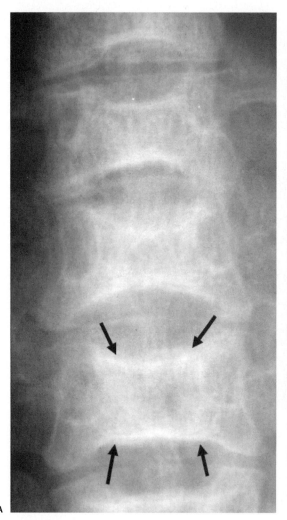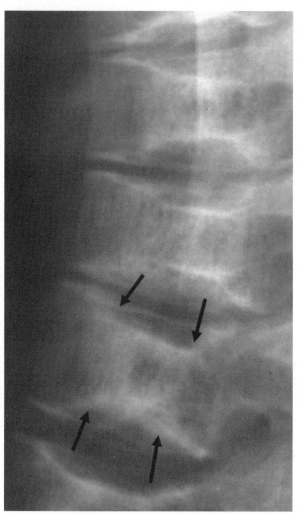

A   B

(A,B) Two views of the thoracolumbar junction show central, squared-off end plate depressions causing an H-shaped vertebra (*arrows*). The trabecular pattern is coarsened.

■ Differential Diagnosis

- **Sickle cell anemia:** An H-shaped vertebra with sclerotic, coarse bony changes in a black patient is diagnostic of sickle cell anemia.
- *Osteoporosis:* The bone mineralization appears normal, and the clinical scenario does not fit. Osteoporotic vertebrae are described as "fish" vertebrae.
- *Gaucher's disease:* The clinical scenario is not consistent with this diagnosis.

■ Essential Facts

- Sickle cell anemia, in which abnormal hemoglobin molecules cause the red blood cells to become rigid and sickle-shaped, is one of a group of conditions known as hemoglobinopathies.
- The consequences are obstruction of the microcirculation, ischemia, and infarction.

- The disease is most prevalent in patients of African origin.
- Infarcts typically occur in the medullary cavities and epiphyses and often are the source of painful bone crises, although they also may be clinically silent and discovered incidentally at radiography.
- H-shaped vertebrae are a consequence of central end plate infarcts.

✔ Pearls & ✘ Pitfalls

- ✔ Compensatory lengthening of the vertebrae adjacent to H-shaped vertebrae may occur; this deformity has been described as "tower" vertebrae.
- ✘ "Fish" vertebrae may occur in sickle cell disease, causing confusion with other metabolic bone diseases.

Case 52

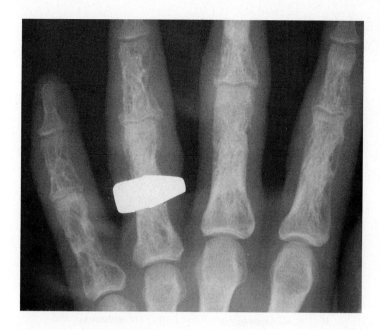

■ Clinical Presentation

A 40-year-old black man presents with mild soft-tissue swelling of the hands.

■ Imaging Findings

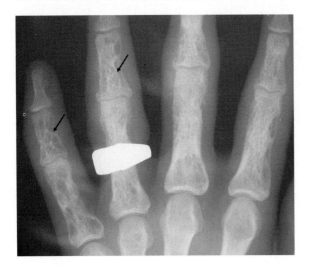

Radiograph of the hand reveals radiolucent lesions in the phalanges with lacelike trabeculation (*arrows*) and mild soft-tissue swelling.

■ Differential Diagnosis

- **Sarcoidosis:** The lacelike trabecular pattern involving multiple phalanges of the hand with associated soft-tissue swelling in a black patient is diagnostic of sarcoidosis.

■ Essential Facts

- Sarcoidosis is a systemic disorder of unknown cause with a wide variety of clinical and radiologic manifestations.
- It is characterized by noncaseating granulomas, which are responsible for the lacelike trabeculation in the hands.
- This disease commonly affects young and middle-aged patients, with a slightly higher prevalence in women and a predilection for African Americans.
- Patients may present with fatigue, weight loss, general malaise, soft-tissue swelling, and cutaneous lesions of the hands and feet.
- Skeletal involvement is seen in ~5% to 10% of patients; the phalanges in the hands and feet are most frequently affected.
- The natural history and prognosis of sarcoidosis are highly variable, and the disease has a tendency to wax and wane.

✔ Pearls & ✘ Pitfalls

- ✔ The articular spaces of the hands are preserved, and there are usually no osseous changes within the metacarpals.
- ✘ Widespread sclerosis may be seen in the vertebrae, mimicking metastasis.

Case 53

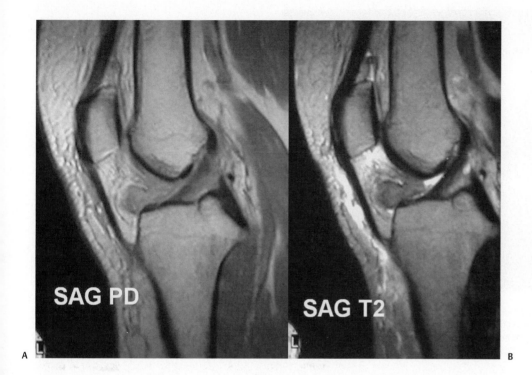

SAG PD

SAG T2

A

B

■ Clinical Presentation

A 25-year-old patient presents with loss of knee extension.

■ Imaging Findings

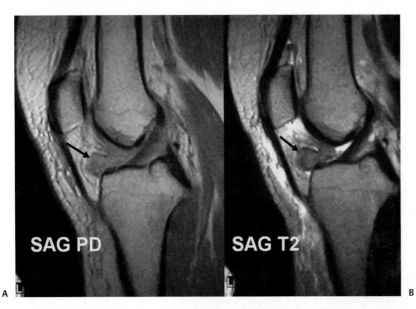

A   B

(A,B) Sagittal proton density- and T2-weighted magnetic resonance (MR) images of the knee show a nodular mass (*arrow*) between the anterior aspect of the lateral femoral condyle and tibia within the anterior intercondylar notch. The lesion, which has intermediate to low signal intensity, abuts the anterior cruciate ligament (ACL).

■ Differential Diagnosis

- *Cyclops lesion:* A lobulated mass with intermediate to low MR signal intensity in this location together with the clinical presentation supports this diagnosis.
- *Focal pigmented villonodular synovitis:* MR ferromagnetic signal loss related to hemosiderin is most typical for this synovial based process.
- *Synovial hemangioma:* Fatty/vascular MR signal characteristics are typically seen with this lesion.

■ Essential Facts

- A cyclops lesion, named because of the bulbous appearance and purplish color resembling an eye at arthroscopy, is comprised of dense fibroconnective vascular tissue.
- This tissue composition gives rise to the intermediate to low MR signal characteristics.
- The lesion results from repetitive microtrauma across the anterior intercondylar soft tissues and is typically recognized after ACL reconstruction.
- However, as in this case, cyclops lesions may occur in the absence of prior ACL reconstruction and be related to chronic ACL tears or subclinical, partially torn ACL fibers.
- Symptoms are related to a mass effect, which blocks extension. MR imaging is the modality of choice for diagnosis.
- The tissue is readily amenable to arthroscopic resection.

✔ Pearls & ✘ Pitfalls

- ✔ An intercondylar mass following ACL repair showing low signal intensity on MR images is characteristic of a cyclops lesion.
- ✘ These lesions may occur in the absence of prior ACL surgery, presenting several years after the inciting traumatic event.

Case 54

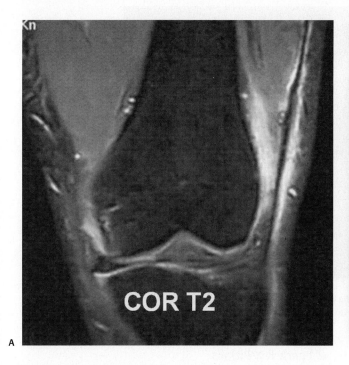

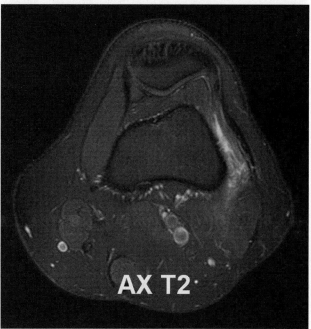

▪ Clinical Presentation

··

A long-distance runner presents with lateral knee pain.

■ Imaging Findings

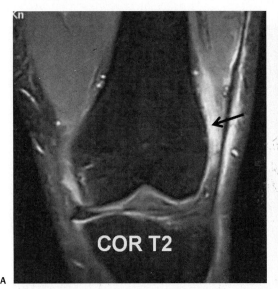
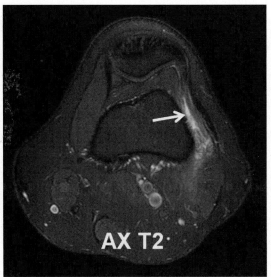

(A,B) Coronal and axial T2-weighted magnetic resonance (MR) images of the knee show a fluid collection (*arrows*) with surrounding inflammation localized between the iliotibial band and femur. No effusion is seen.

■ Differential Diagnosis

• ***Iliotibial band friction syndrome:*** Focal fluid and/or inflammation between the iliotibial band and lateral femoral epicondyle in a runner is diagnostic of this syndrome.

■ Essential Facts

• Iliotibial band friction syndrome is an overuse phenomenon related to abnormal contact between the iliotibial band and the lateral femoral epicondyle during repetitive flexion and extension of the knee.
• The iliotibial band is formed proximally by the fascia of the gluteus maximus and gluteus medius and the tensor fasciae latae.
• Distally, the iliotibial band extends below the joint to insert on Gerdy's tubercle of the tibia.
• Iliotibial band friction syndrome is seen in long-distance runners, cyclists, and football players.
• This syndrome is a common cause of lateral knee pain that may be confused with lateral meniscal tears, lateral collateral ligament injuries, or injuries to the insertion of the biceps femoris or popliteus muscles.
• MR images demonstrate increased signal intensity or a fluid collection deep to the iliotibial band.
• Frequently, the band is thickened, with intermediate signal intensity.

✔ Pearls & ✘ Pitfalls

✔ Mild subcortical edema may be seen along the posterior lateral epicondyle of the femur.
✘ A localized effusion within the lateral suprapatellar bursa may be mistaken for this process.

Case 55

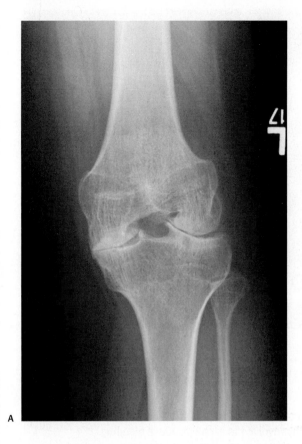

A

▨ Clinical Presentation

A 25-year-old patient presents with a history of a bleeding diathesis.

Further Work-up

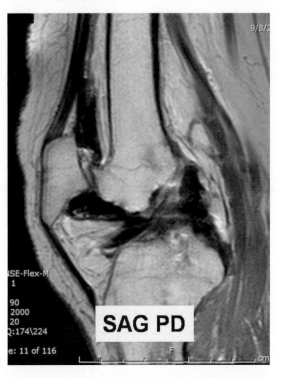

SAG PD

B

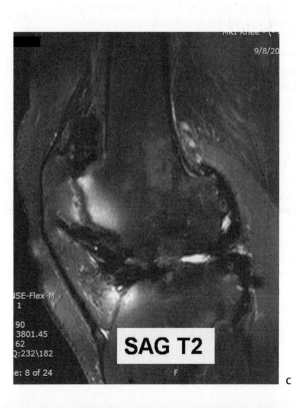

SAG T2

C

■ Imaging Findings

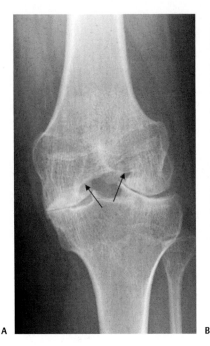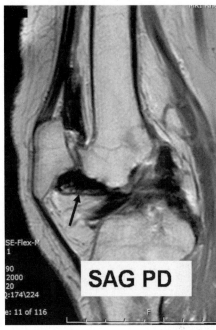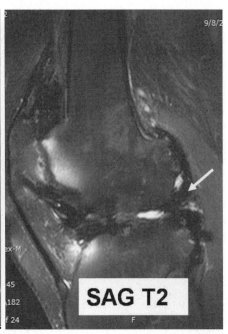

A   B   C

(A) Radiograph of the knee shows osteopenia with enlargement of the epiphyses, narrowing of the joint spaces, and a widened intercondylar notch (*black arrows*). Squaring is seen in the inferior patellar margin. **(B,C)** Sagittal proton density- and T2-weighted magnetic resonance (MR) images show uniformly thickened synovial tissue with low signal intensity (*arrows*) related to hemosiderin deposits.

■ Differential Diagnosis

- **Hemophilic arthropathy:** The clinical presentation, the radiographic findings of a widened intercondylar notch, epiphyseal overgrowth, a squared patella, and the low synovial signal intensity on MR images are characteristic of this arthropathy.
- *Pigmented villonodular synovitis:* This is a monarticular disease that tends to exhibit nodular/lobular synovial thickening with low signal intensity.
- *Juvenile rheumatoid arthritis:* MR findings of this disease include synovitis in the form of increased T2 signal intensity within thickened synovial tissues.

■ Essential Facts

- Hemophilia is a bleeding disorder related to a deficiency/disorder of clotting factors.
- It may be associated with repeated bleeding into the synovial joints and subsequent arthropathic changes.
- Episodes of bleeding tend to recur in the same joint and cause synovial hyperplasia, chronic inflammatory changes, fibrosis, and siderosis of the synovial membrane.
- The hemosiderin deposits account for the MR findings of low signal intensity within the synovium.
- In descending order, the knee, ankle, elbow, and shoulder are the most commonly affected joints.

- Bilateral involvement is common, although a single joint is usually involved in each episode of bleeding.
- Hemophilic arthropathy most often occurs in the 1st or 2nd decade of life.

✔ Pearls & ✘ Pitfalls

- ✔ A factor distinguishing juvenile rheumatoid arthritis from hemophilic arthropathy is involvement of the hands/feet and spine with the former.
- ✘ Hemarthrosis after trauma is common in this age group.

Case 56

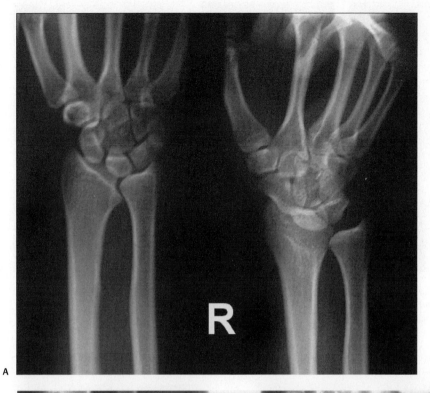

A

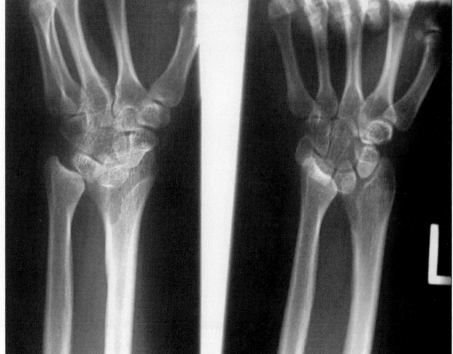

B

■ Clinical Presentation

A 25-year-old woman presents with bilateral wrist deformities and decreased range of motion.

■ Imaging Findings

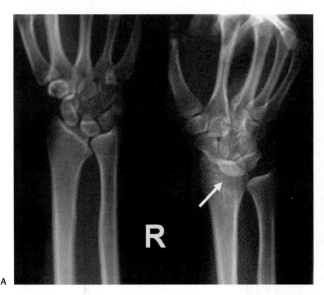
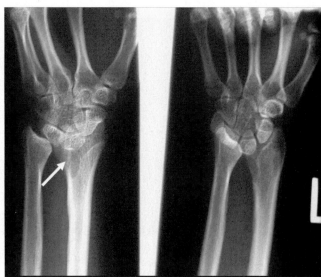

A   B

(A,B) Radiographs of the wrists show deformities bilaterally. There is increased ulnar inclination of the distal radial articular surfaces, which display a triangular configuration. Hypoplastic-appearing changes along the medial margins of the distal radii are seen. Increased lucency is seen over the ulnar aspects of the distal radii (*arrows*).

■ Differential Diagnosis

- **Madelung deformity:** A bilateral abnormal configuration of the distal radii, which show underdevelopment along the ulnar margins and a triangular shape, is strongly associated with this deformity.

■ Essential Facts

- Madelung deformity is a primary or secondary phenomenon associated with underdevelopment of the medial margin of the distal radius.
- Consequently, a medial slant occurs along the distal radial surface such that the radius resembles a triangle, with medial lucent changes seen on radiographs.
- The causes are multiple and include bone dysplasias (dyschondrosteosis), Turner syndrome, osteochondromatosis, trauma, and infection.
- Women are affected more commonly, presenting with pain and decreased range of motion.

✔ Pearls & ✗ Pitfalls

- ✔ Madelung deformity is more commonly bilateral with an asymmetric pattern of deformity.
- ✗ The increased lucency seen over the ulnar aspect of the distal radius may be confused with a bony lesion.

Case 57

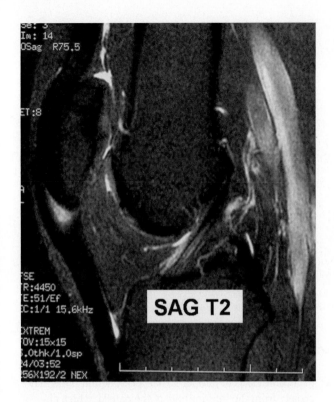

◼ Clinical Presentation

A 38-year-old recreational athlete presents with knee pain.

■ Imaging Findings

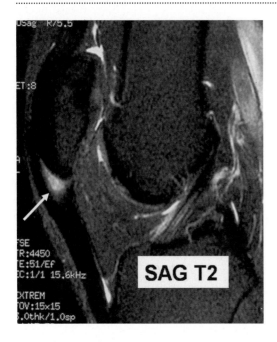

Sagittal T2-weighted magnetic resonance (MR) image of the knee shows increased signal intensity (*arrow*) in the proximal patellar tendon with expansion of the tendon.

■ Differential Diagnosis

• **Jumper's knee:** The patient's presentation combined with enlargement, edema, and increased T2 signal intensity in the proximal patellar tendon is characteristic of this diagnosis.

■ Essential Facts

• Jumper's knee is proximal patellar tendonosis that is associated with repetitive overloading of the extensor mechanism of the knee.
• The injury occurs in sports that require explosive jumping movements, such as basketball, volleyball, and soccer.
• Patients present with pain at the proximal insertion of the patellar tendon.
• This typically occurs during the adolescent years and is seen more often in boys.
• The MR signal abnormality within the tendon represents microtears, which continue unless the aggravating activity is stopped for a period of time.

✔ Pearls & ✘ Pitfalls

✔ In chronic cases of jumper's knee, protuberant bone may project from the inferior pole of the patella, which appears to be elongated.
✘ Sinding-Larsen-Johansson disease, an osteochondrosis of the distal patellar pole at the insertion of the patellar tendon, may be confused with this diagnosis.

Case 58

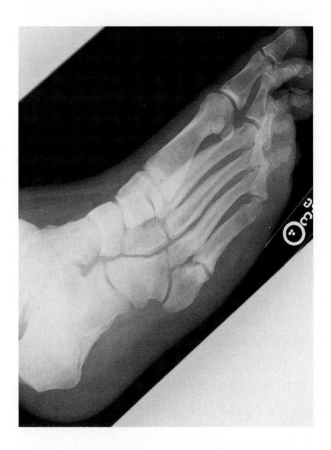

■ Clinical Presentation

A 30-year-old man presents for 6-month follow-up of a fracture.

■ Imaging Findings

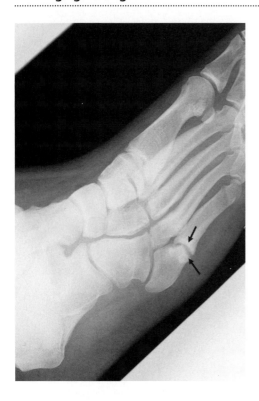

Radiograph of the foot shows a fracture extending through the proximal diaphysis of the fifth metatarsal. Sclerosis and callus (*arrows*) line the margins of the fracture without osseous bridging across the fracture defect.

■ Differential Diagnosis

- ***Non-union Jones fracture:*** A transverse fracture through the junction of the proximal diaphysis and metaphysis of the fifth metatarsal is a Jones fracture. The absence of bridging callus is consistent with non-union.
- *Dancer's fracture:* This is an oblique, minimally displaced avulsion fracture at the base of the fifth metatarsal.
- *March fracture:* This is a stress fracture typically seen in the second and third metatarsals that is related to chronic overload.

■ Essential Facts

- A Jones fracture is a fracture of the proximal diaphysis of the fifth metatarsal that is distal to the metatarsal tuberosity.
- It results from either direct or indirect forces.
- The importance of this fracture is that aggressive treatment is required because of the high prevalence of non-union related to focal bony hypovascularity.
- The absence of weight bearing is typically required for appropriate healing.

✔ Pearls & ✘ Pitfalls

- ✔ Jones fractures typically rebreak if not appropriately immobilized.
- ✘ A Jones fracture is commonly confused with a dancer's fracture given the proximity of the two types of injury.

Case 59

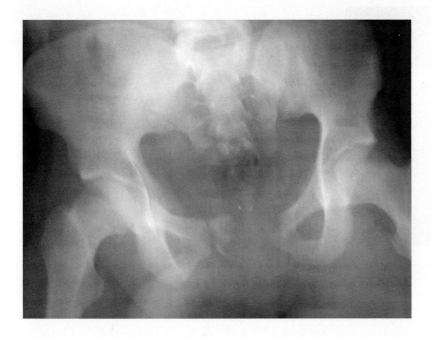

▪ Clinical Presentation

The patient has been injured in a motor vehicle crash.

■ Imaging Findings

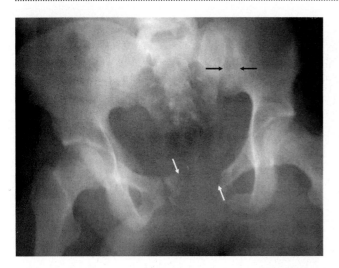

Radiograph of the pelvis shows a vertically oriented fracture through the left pubic bone with marked offset across the fracture defect (white arrows). Significant diastasis of the left sacroiliac (SI) joint (*black arrows*) is seen.

■ Differential Diagnosis

• **Open-book pelvic fracture:** Significant splaying/widening across a vertically oriented fracture of the left pubic bone with associated SI joint diastasis is diagnostic of an open-book pelvic fracture.

■ Essential Facts

• Open-book pelvic fractures are the second most common type of pelvic fracture, the first being lateral compression fractures.
• Open-book fractures result when an anteroposterior force on the anterior pelvis distracts the pubic symphysis and SI joints.
• Alternatively, depending on the direct anterior force applied, a distracted vertical fracture of the pubic bone may replace the diastasis of the pubic symphysis.
• This fracture pattern relates to the application of force to a ring structure resulting in two points of failure in the ring.
• Arterial hemorrhage is frequently associated with this injury. Specifically, the superior gluteal and internal pudendal arteries may be injured.
• Additionally, urethral injuries are common, particularly in male crash victims.
• For these reasons, computed tomography of the abdomen and pelvis must be performed, with particular attention to the iliac arteries and the urogenital system.

✔ Pearls & ✗ Pitfalls

✔ Arterial hemorrhage is frequently associated with this injury.
✗ Radiographs often fail to display nondisplaced sacral and pubic fractures.

Case 60

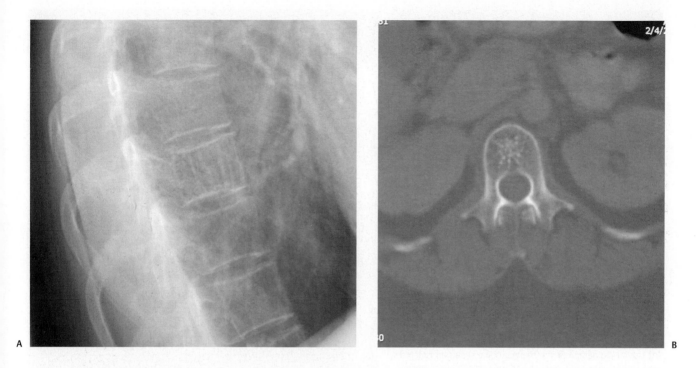

A   B

■ Clinical Presentation

An abnormality is seen on a chest radiograph and a computed tomographic (CT) scan.

■ Imaging Findings

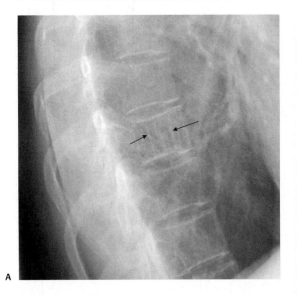

A

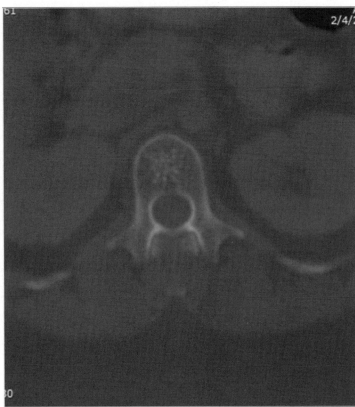

B

(A) Lateral radiograph of the thoracic spine shows an isolated area with a coarsened vertical trabecular pattern resembling corduroy (*arrows*) within a thoracic vertebral body. **(B)** Axial CT scan through this level shows a "polka dot" appearance of the trabeculae.

■ Differential Diagnosis

- **Vertebral hemangioma:** An isolated vertebral body demonstrating vertically oriented, coarsened trabeculae in a "corduroy" pattern is diagnostic of a vertebral hemangioma.
- *Paget's disease:* This process typically causes horizontal trabecular condensation and vertebral body enlargement.
- *Rugger jersey spine:* Thick, horizontal sclerotic bands at the end plates of vertebral bodies are typical of this diagnosis.

■ Essential Facts

- Vertebral hemangiomas are very common, accounting for 28% of all skeletal hemangiomas.
- Compensatory trabecular thickening occurs as a result of the overgrowth of fatty vascular tissue.
- The thoracic spine is the most common location.
- Hemangiomas may be multiple in one third of cases.
- Patients may have neurologic symptoms if the process extends into and expands the posterior elements.
- However, most vertebral hemangiomas are incidentally discovered and require no treatment.

✔ Pearls & ✘ Pitfalls

- ✔ Magnetic resonance imaging typically shows bright signal on T1- and T2-weighted sequences that is related to the fat content.
- ✘ Irregular, focal radiolucent areas within a vertebral body may be seen on radiographs, simulating a malignant neoplasm.

Case 61

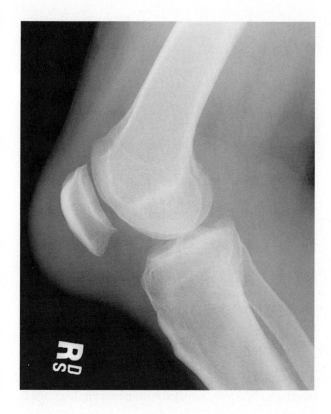

■ Clinical Presentation

A 45-year-old construction worker presents with knee pain and fullness.

■ Imaging Findings

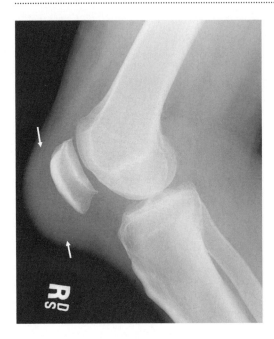

A lateral radiograph of the knee shows a nonmineralized soft-tissue mass (arrows) anterior to the patella with mild patellofemoral arthritic changes.

■ Differential Diagnosis

- **Prepatellar bursitis:** Focal soft-tissue swelling anterior to the patella in a manual laborer without other systemic signs or symptoms is characteristic of prepatellar bursitis.
- *Septic bursitis:* The clinical scenario does not support infection.
- *Inflammation-induced bursitis:* The absence of soft-tissue/bursal calcifications and/or arthropathic changes excludes an inflammatory response related to gout or rheumatoid arthritis.

■ Essential Facts

- Prepatellar bursitis (housemaid's knee or carpet layer's knee) is inflammation in the prepatellar bursa, which is located anteriorly between the patella and subcutaneous tissues. The bursa becomes inflamed and hypertrophic in response to minor repetitive injury, such as that sustained while working on one's hands and knees. The typical patient presents with a chronically enlarged prepatellar bursa and focal pain and swelling.

■ Other Imaging Findings

- Magnetic resonance imaging (MRI) reveals a focal fluid collection anterior to the patella demonstrating high signal intensity on T2-weighted images.

✔ Pearls & ✘ Pitfalls

- ✔ Degenerative arthritic changes localized to the patello-femoral joint commonly coexist with prepatellar bursitis.
- ✘ Hemorrhage may coexist with the inflammation, appearing as a heterogeneous mass on MRI and complicating the diagnosis.

Case 62

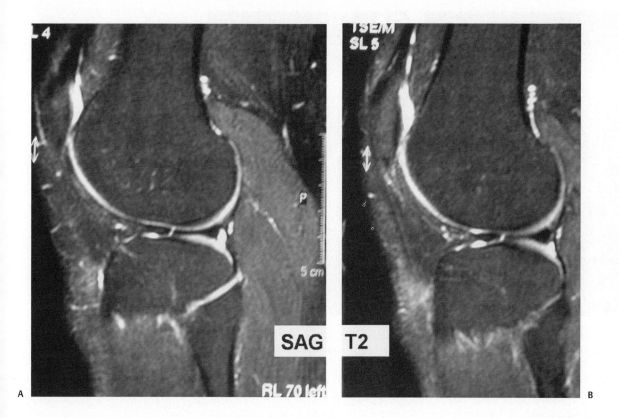

Clinical Presentation

The patient presents with lateral joint line knee pain and normal findings on radiographs of the knee.

■ **Imaging Findings**

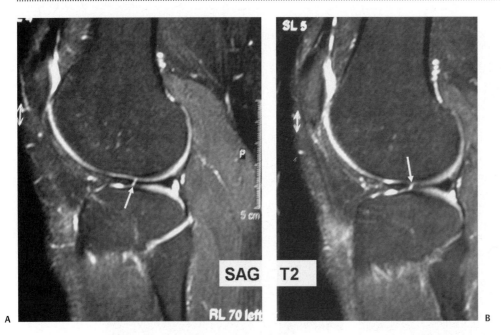

(A,B) Sagittal T2-weighted fat-saturated images of the knee demonstrate a vertically oriented cleft of increased T2 signal intensity extending through the anterior horn of the lateral meniscus (*arrows*) and opening onto the femoral and tibial articular surfaces. This defect is perpendicular to the circumferential semicircular axis of the lateral meniscus.

■ **Differential Diagnosis**

• **Radial meniscal tear:** Abnormally increased T2 signal intensity extending to the meniscal surface and oriented perpendicular to the circumferential axis of the meniscus is diagnostic of a radial meniscal tear.

■ **Essential Facts**

• Radial meniscal tears occur in a plane perpendicular to the circumferential axis of the meniscus and tibial plateau.
• These tears traverse the circumferential collagen fibers and may result in division of the meniscus into two separate pieces.
• Radial meniscal tears account for ~14% of all meniscal tears.
• These tears disrupt the distribution of hoop stresses associated with weight bearing and result in pain.
• Radial meniscal tears usually cannot be repaired.

✔ **Pearls & ✗ Pitfalls**

✔ The majority of radial meniscal tears occur in posterior meniscal horns. A marching cleft may be seen at the junction of the posterior horn and body, in which the tear appears to "move" across the meniscus on successive images.
✗ Small radial meniscal tears can be overlooked if they appear as a blur on a single image.

Case 63

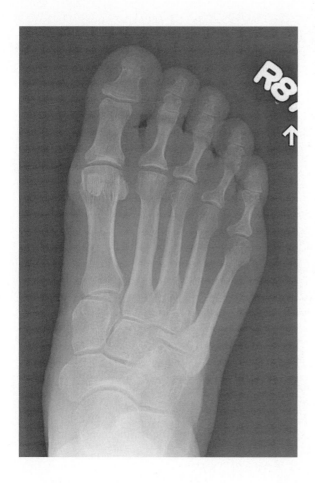

◼ Clinical Presentation

A 30-year-old woman presents with chronic pain in the right forefoot.

■ Imaging Findings

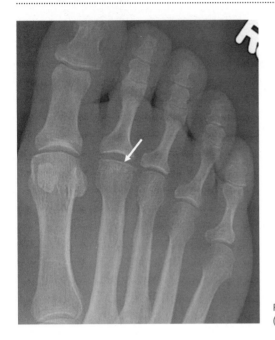

Radiograph of the foot shows sclerosis and flattening of the head of the second metatarsal (*arrow*) with mild arthritic changes affecting this joint.

■ Differential Diagnosis

- **Freiberg's disease:** Features of avascular necrosis, including heterogeneous density with deformity/flattening localized to the head of the second metatarsal and secondary osteoarthrosis, are characteristic of this diagnosis.

■ Essential Facts

- Freiberg's disease, or osteonecrosis of the head of the second metatarsal, seems to result from repetitive trauma and vascular compromise with subsequent osteochondral fracture through the distal articular surface of the metatarsal.
- The second metatarsal is the most commonly involved bone, followed by the third metatarsal.
- This disorder is seen most often in athletic adolescent girls, who present with focal pain and tenderness.
- High-heeled shoes have been implicated as a causative factor in older women.

■ Other Imaging Findings

- Findings on magnetic resonance imaging include decreased signal intensity in the head of the metatarsal on T1-weighted images and increased signal intensity on corresponding T2-weighted and short time inversion recovery (STIR) images.

✔ Pearls & ✗ Pitfalls

- ✔ This disease process may be bilateral in up to 10% of patients.
- ✗ Initially, radiographic findings are often negative.

Case 64

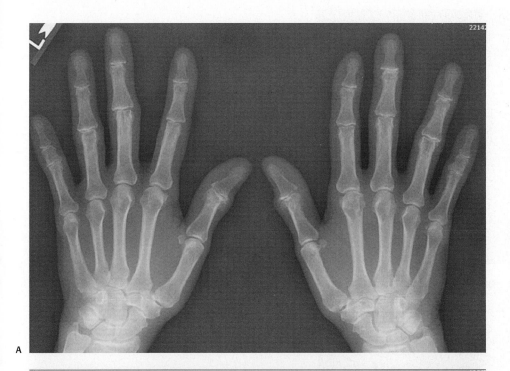

A

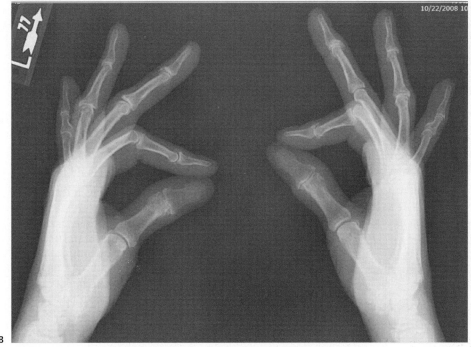

B

▪ Clinical Presentation
....

A 63-year-old woman presents with chronic recurring hand pain.

■ Imaging Findings

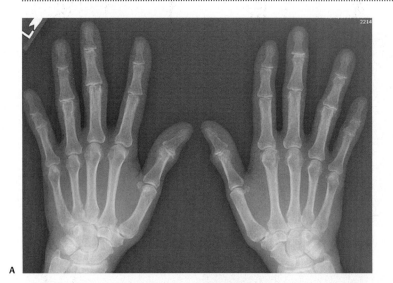

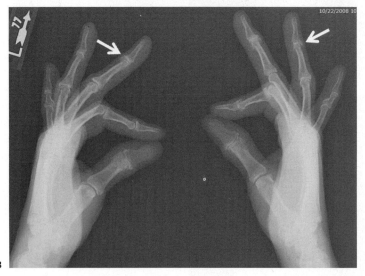

(A,B) Radiographs of the hands show narrowing of the interphalangeal (IP) joint space, subchondral sclerosis, and osteophyte formation (*arrows*). No erosions, subluxations, or osteopenia are seen.

■ Differential Diagnosis

- **Osteoarthrosis:** Osteophytes, sclerosis of bone, and loss of joint space predominantly in the IP joints of the hands suggest osteoarthrosis.
- *Erosive osteoarthritis:* The absence of subarticular erosions excludes this diagnosis.
- *Rheumatoid arthritis:* The absence of symmetric, deforming, erosive articular changes and osteopenia makes this an unlikely diagnosis.

■ Essential Facts

- Osteoarthrosis results from damage to the articular cartilage caused by repetitive microtrauma that occurs throughout the life process.
- It tends to involve specific synovial joints during specific decades of a person's life and depends in part on the patient's level of physical activity.
- Osteoarthrosis characteristically involves the IP joints of the hands after the 4th or 5th decade of life; it is related in part to the degree of use and overuse.
- Involvement of the metacarpophalangeal joints is not infrequently associated with osteoarthrosis of the IP joints, although metacarpophalangeal involvement is usually less severe.
- The presence of osteophytes with sclerosis of bone and the absence of inflammatory features such as erosions suggest this diagnosis.
- As the joint space narrows, the osteophytes may become larger.

✔ Pearls & ✗ Pitfalls

- ✔ Another typical site of osteoarthrosis is the first carpometacarpal joint, where it often begins after the fifth decade of life. This is attributed in part to stresses related to the constant use of opposing thumbs or joint laxity.
- ✗ Occasionally, an inflammatory component of osteoarthrosis can develop about the hands and cause an appearance similar to that of erosive osteoarthritis.

Case 65

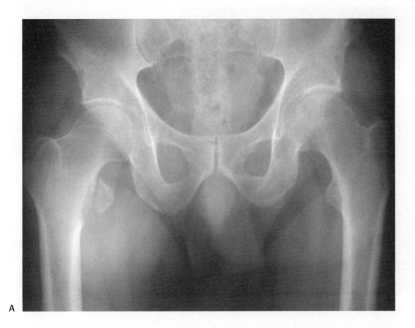

A

■ Clinical Presentation

A 60-year-old man presents with atraumatic pain in the right groin.

Further Work-up

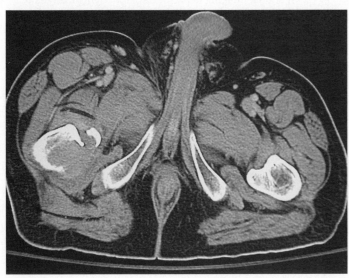

B

■ Imaging Findings

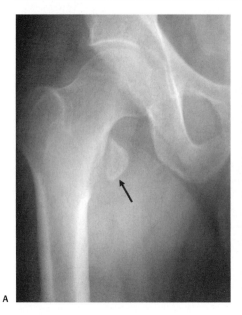
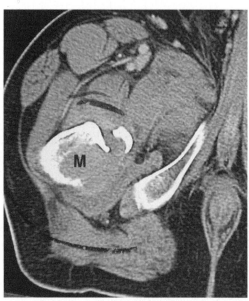

A   B

(A) Frontal radiograph of the pelvis shows an avulsion fracture (*arrow*) of the right lesser trochanter. **(B)** Axial computed tomographic (CT) scan through the fracture site shows an intramedullary soft-tissue mass (*M*) at the site of the lesser trochanter.

■ Differential Diagnosis

• *Pathologic avulsion fracture of the lesser trochanter:*
An atraumatic avulsion fracture of the lesser trochanter in an older adult with CT demonstration of an underlying intramedullary soft-tissue mass is pathognomonic for a pathologic fracture.

■ Essential Facts

• Avulsion fractures of the lesser trochanter are related to traction from the iliopsoas muscle and tendon.
• This is a rare traumatic avulsion fracture in the young athlete.
• An adult presenting with this fracture, particularly an older adult without a history of trauma, is highly likely to have an underlying malignancy.
• The exact reason for this is unknown.
• The most common underlying lesion is a metastasis.

✔ Pearls & ✘ Pitfalls

✔ Any adult with an atraumatic avulsion fracture of the lesser trochanter must be further evaluated with cross-sectional imaging to exclude an underlying malignant process.
✘ Radiography often fails to display the underlying osseous lesion at the time of presentation.

Case 66

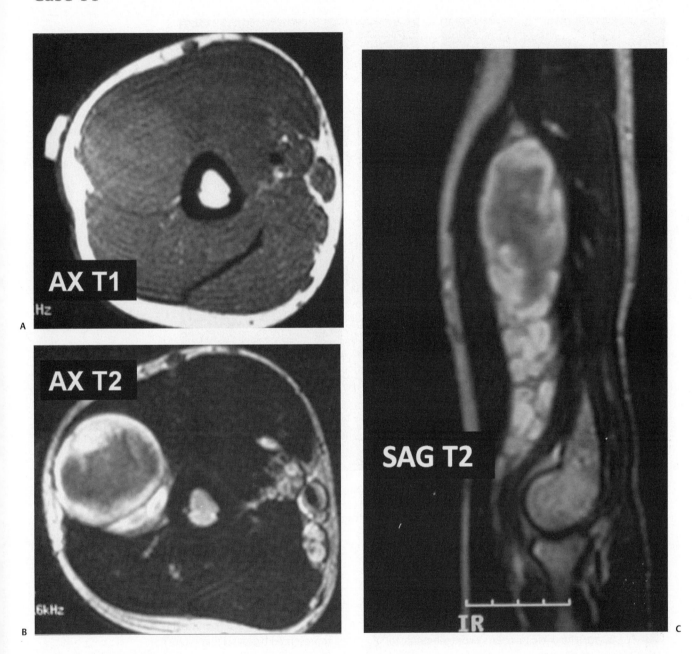

A

B

C

Clinical Presentation

A 30-year-old man presents with scattered areas of skin discoloration and soft-tissue masses along the right arm.

■ Imaging Findings

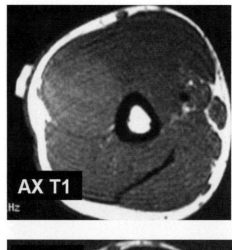

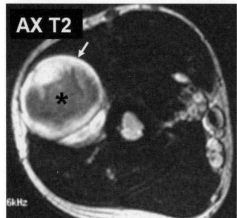

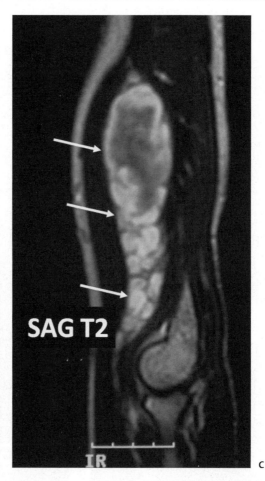

(A–C) Magnetic resonance (MR) images of the right arm reveal convoluted multinodular masses and thickening (*long arrows*) along the expected course of the radial nerve. The axial T2-weighted MR image shows high signal intensity peripherally (*short arrow*) with low signal intensity centrally (*asterisk*), the "target sign."

■ Differential Diagnosis

- **Plexiform neurofibroma:** The history of skin discoloration (café au lait spots) in combination with replacement of the radial nerve by a plexiform mass displaying a "target sign" on T2-weighted MR images is pathognomonic for a plexiform neurofibroma.

■ Essential Facts

- Neurogenic neoplasms account for ~10% to 12% of all benign soft-tissue neoplasms.
- Neurofibroma most commonly affects patients 20 to 30 years of age and shows no sex predilection.
- Three types of neurofibromas are classically described: localized, diffuse, and plexiform (associated with neurofibromatosis type 1).
- A plexiform neurofibroma represents diffuse intraneural neoplastic overgrowth of a long nerve segment with tortuous expansion of its branches.

- The gross appearance has been described as a "bag of worms."
- The "target sign" on T2-weighted MR images is the consequence of peripheral myxomatous tissue, represented by high signal intensity, enclosing central fibrous tissue, represented by low signal intensity.
- Plexiform neurofibroma may be accompanied by osseous hypertrophy related to chronic hyperemia.
- Because of the large size of many of these lesions, surgical resection is often incomplete, so that recurrences are frequent.
- Transformation to a malignant peripheral nerve sheath tumor is the most feared complication.

✔ Pearls & ✘ Pitfalls

- ✔ The "target sign" on T2-weighted MR images combined with a multiplicity of lesions having nodular morphology is pathognomonic for this entity.
- ✘ The differentiation of schwannomas from neurofibromas and of benign from malignant nerve sheath tumors can be problematic.

Case 67

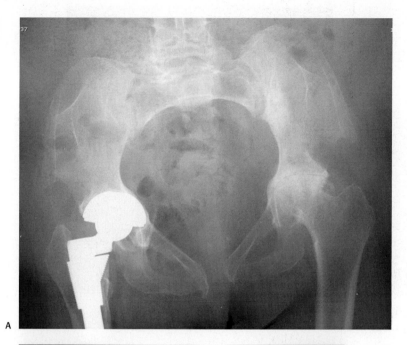

A

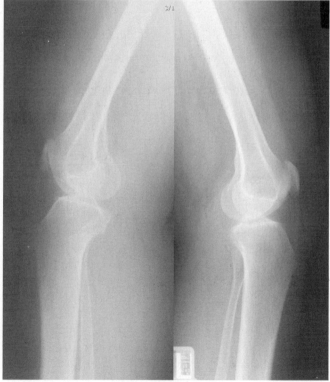

B

■ Clinical Presentation

A 66-year-old woman presents with bilateral hip and knee pain.

■ Imaging Findings

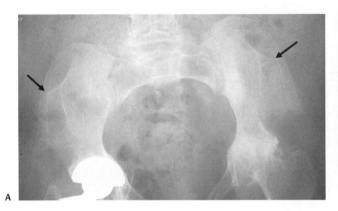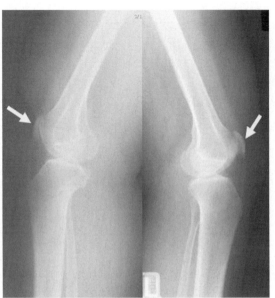

A   B

(A,B) Radiographs of the pelvis and knees show posterior iliac horns (*black arrows*) and hypoplastic patellae (*white arrows*) bilaterally. Dysplasia of the iliac wings is noted. Severe osteoarthritic change of the left hip is present.

■ Differential Diagnosis

- **Fong disease:** Radiographic findings of hypoplastic patellae combined with posterior iliac horns is pathognomonic for Fong disease.

■ Essential Facts

- Fong disease, also known as hereditary osteo-onycho-dysplasia or nail-patella syndrome, consists of a clinical pentad of nail dysplasia, hypoplastic or absent patellae, dislocation of the radial heads, iliac horns, and renal dysplasia.
- The pattern of inheritance of this syndrome is autosomal-dominant, and it manifests clinically in the 2nd or 3rd decade.
- The smooth bony outgrowths arising from the posterior iliac bones are asymptomatic and frequently palpable.
- The horns are located at the site of attachment of the gluteus medius muscle.

✔ Pearls & ✗ Pitfalls

- ✔ Bilateral posterior iliac bony outgrowths are diagnostic of this disease.
- ✗ Twenty percent of patients may not have iliac horns.

Case 68

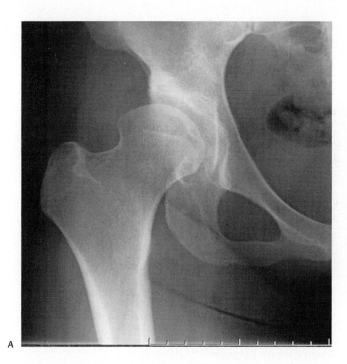

A

■ Clinical Presentation

A 40-year-old woman presents with pain/clicking in the right hip.

Further Work-up

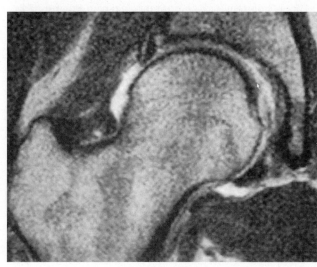

B

■ Imaging Findings

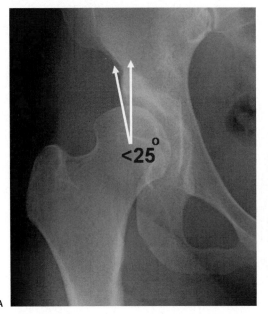
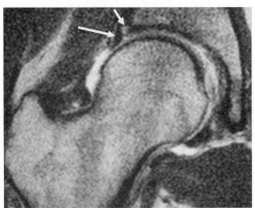

(A) Frontal radiograph of the right hip shows deficient acetabular coverage of the femoral head. The center–edge angle is < 25 degrees (*arrows*). Degenerative sclerosis lines the superior acetabulum. **(B)** Coronal magnetic resonance (MR) imaging with intra-articular contrast depicts abnormally increased signal intensity (*short arrow*) at the interface between the acetabular rim and the labrum of the hip (*long arrow*).

■ Differential Diagnosis

• **Developmental hip dysplasia with labral tear:** Deficient acetabular coverage of the femoral head with a center–edge angle of < 25 degrees represents developmental hip dysplasia. Increased MR imaging signal intensity from intra-articular contrast at the interface between the labrum of the hip and the underlying acetabular rim represents a labral tear.

■ Essential Facts

• In developmental hip dysplasia, the femoral head is only partially covered by the acetabulum.
• The center–edge angle is used to quantify acetabular coverage of the femoral head.
• The angle is formed by two lines. Each originates at the center of the femoral head, with one line extending vertically and the second extending to the lateral acetabulum.
• Coverage of the femoral head is considered adequate if the angle measures ≥ 25 degrees.
• The cause of this condition is controversial. It most likely develops in utero and is related to the fetal position.
• Patients are at increased risk for labral tears.
• Labral tears result from the increased weight-bearing role of the labrum, which is a consequence of deficient acetabular coverage of the femoral head.

• The possibility of a pathologic labral condition should be considered in individuals with developmental dysplasia of the hip whose pain is disproportionate to the radiographic changes.
• The process is typically unilateral.
• Patients present with anterior inguinal pain, painful clicking, transient locking, and instability of the hip.
• The condition is seen more commonly in female patients.

✔ Pearls & ✗ Pitfalls

✔ Developmental hip dysplasia is associated with labral tears along the anterosuperior quadrant of the acetabulum.
✗ Neuromuscular diseases may mimic a developmentally dysplastic hip radiographically.

Case 69

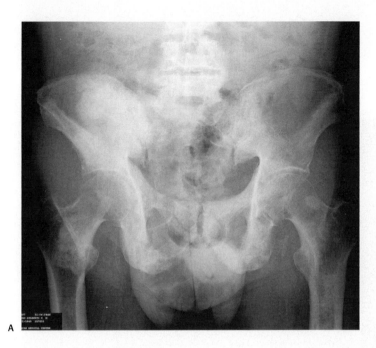

A

■ Clinical Presentation

A 70-year-old man presents with buttock pain.

Further Work-up

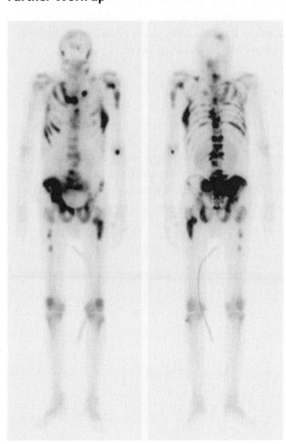

B

■ Imaging Findings

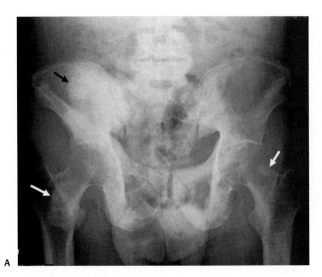

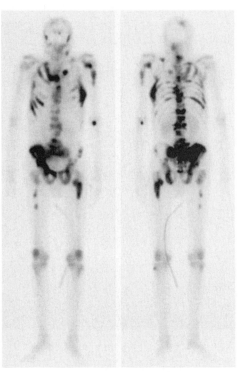

A   B

(A) Anteroposterior view of the pelvis demonstrates widespread sclerotic foci (*arrows*) within the pelvic bones and femora. **(B)** Bone scan demonstrates multiple focal areas of increased radionuclide uptake in the pelvic bones, femora, spine, scapulae, skull, humeri, and ribs.

■ Differential Diagnosis

- *Osteoblastic prostate metastasis:* Replacement of large areas of bone by irregular, patchy, dense lesions showing multifocal uptake on bone scan in an elderly man is diagnostic of osteoblastic prostate metastasis.
- *Paget's disease:* The irregular, patchy distribution of sclerotic bone and lack of trabecular coarsening do not favor this nonmalignant process.
- *Osteopoikilosis:* The multifocal, patchy bony involvement lacking a periarticular distribution does not favor osteopoikilosis.

■ Essential Facts

- The skeleton is the most common site of hematogenous metastases of prostate cancer.
- Metastases to bone can be found in 85% of patients dying of this disease.
- Osteoblastic metastases account for the majority of these skeletal lesions.
- The bone findings may completely reverse after androgen ablation therapy, although a paradoxical, transient increase in skeletal osteoblastic activity (flare effect) may occur after orchiectomy or androgen blockade.

- Because of the high sensitivity of radionuclide scintigraphy in detecting osteoblastic metastases, bone scan has replaced the skeletal survey in the evaluation of patients with suspected metastases to bone.

✔ Pearls & ✗ Pitfalls

- ✔ Osteoblastic prostate metastases predominate in the axial skeleton.
- ✗ Plain radiographs are not very sensitive for detecting early metastases to bone because a change in bone density of 30%–50% typically must occur before metastases can be seen.

Case 70

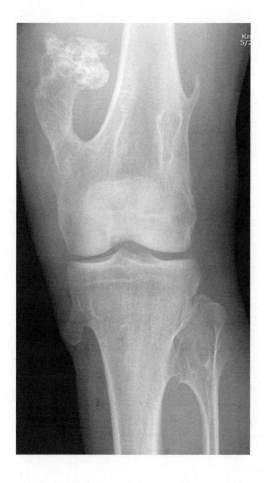

■ Clinical Presentation

A patient presents with a lower extremity deformity and a family history of abnormal bones.

■ Imaging Findings

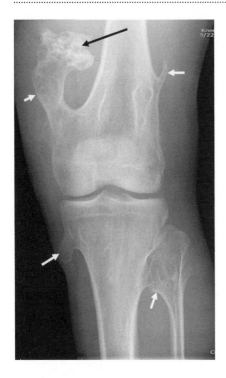

Radiograph of the left knee show multiple bony protuberances (*white arrows*) extending from the distal femur and proximal tibia and fibula. The lesions are continuous with the cortical and medullary bone and point away from the knee joint. No soft-tissue mass is seen. Calcifications over the femoral lesion (*black arrow*) are seen.

■ Differential Diagnosis

- *Osteochondromatosis:* Multiple bony outgrowths continuous with the cortical and medullary bone, one of which contains a calcified cartilage cap, are pathognomonic for osteochondromatosis.

■ Essential Facts

- Osteochondromatosis (also referred to as multiple hereditary exostoses) is an autosomal-dominant syndrome.
- Patients exhibit multiple pedunculated or sessile bony protuberances lined by a cartilage cap with or without chondroid calcifications.
- Depending on the genetic variation, these lesions may be bilateral or unilateral in distribution.
- The long bones of the lower extremity are most frequently affected.
- The skull is the only bone that is spared in this condition.
- Malignant transformation is seen in 3% to 5% of patients and is manifested by continued growth of lesions and a hyaline cartilage cap with a thickness of > 1.5 cm.
- The condition is usually diagnosed before the age of 12 years because of the bony deformities.
- Boys are affected more commonly.
- Magnetic resonance imaging is the best radiologic modality for visualizing the effect of the lesion on surrounding structures and evaluating the hyaline cartilage cap.

✔ Pearls & ✘ Pitfalls

- ✔ The lesions of osteochondromatosis are typically sessile. Centrally located osteochondromas about the pelvis, hips, and shoulders are more prone to undergo malignant transformation.
- ✘ Evaluation of the cartilage cap may be limited by surrounding inflammation and/or adventitial bursal formation.

Case 71

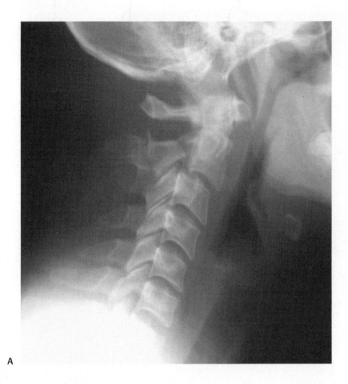

A

■ Clinical Presentation

A patient presents with neck pain after a motor vehicle collision.

Further Work-up

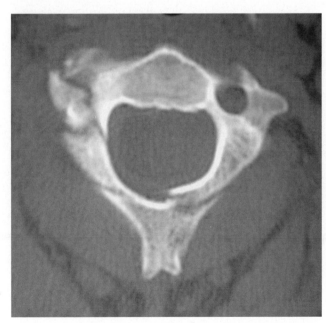

B

■ Imaging Findings

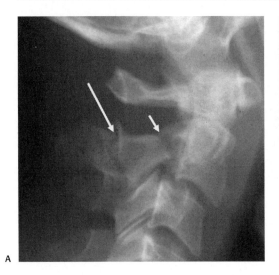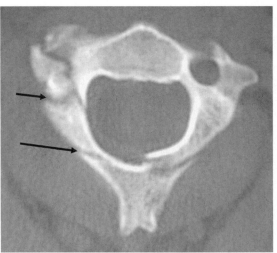

A   B

(A) Lateral radiograph of the cervical spine shows fractures through the lamina (long arrow) and pars interarticularis (*short arrow*) of C2 with associated C2-C3 anterolisthesis. **(B)** Axial computed tomographic (CT) scan through C2 shows a fracture line extending through the right pars interarticularis (*short arrow*) with extension into the right vertebral foramen. A laminar fracture (*long arrow*) is also seen.

■ Differential Diagnosis

- *Hangman's fracture:* Fractures through the laminae or pedicles of C2 associated with C2-C3 anterolisthesis are characteristic of this injury.

■ Essential Facts

- A hangman's fracture may be unilateral or bilateral. Fractures through the C2 laminae or pedicles are associated with anterolisthesis of the body of C2 on C3.
- A direct blow to the face with hyperextension is the typical mechanism. This is the second most common C2 fracture.
- Subsequent separation of the body and posterior arch of C2 allows decompression of the spinal cord.
- These are considered unstable fractures.
- CT is recommended to optimally demonstrate the location and orientation of the fracture planes.

✔ Pearls & ✗ Pitfalls

- ✔ Widening of the C2-C3 disk space and bilateral interfacetal dislocation may be seen, indicating a more severe injury.
- ✗ An atypical variant of this injury, which may be less evident on radiographs, involves the posterior vertebral body of C2.

Case 72

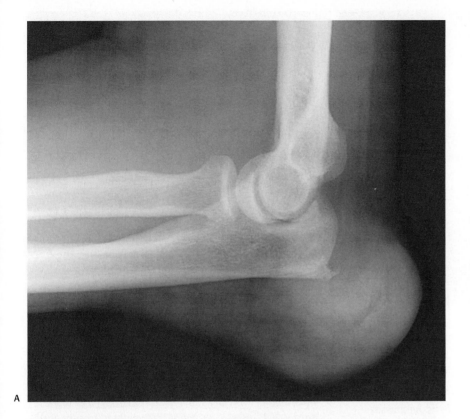

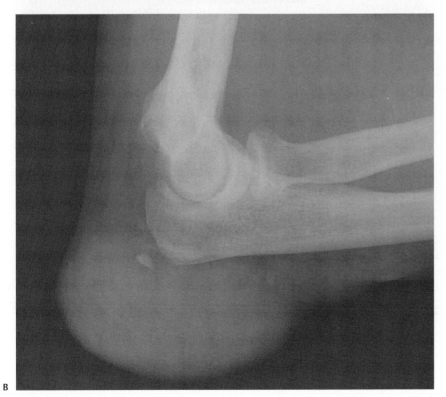

■ Clinical Presentation

A 55-year-old man presents with arthralgias and bilateral elbow masses.

■ Imaging Findings

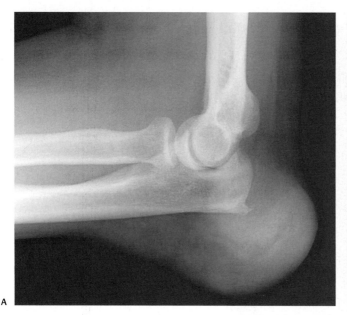
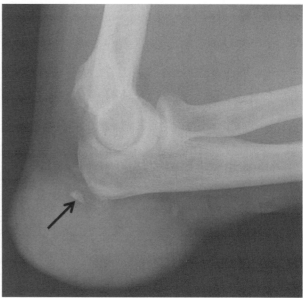

A   B

(A,B) Lateral radiographs of the elbows show large, radiodense, faintly mineralized soft-tissue masses in the expected region of the olecranon bursae. Bony fragments are noted on the left (*arrow*). The joint spaces are maintained, and no erosions are seen. Olecranon enthesophytes are present.

■ Differential Diagnosis

- ***Tophaceous gout:*** Dense, mineralized soft-tissue masses involving the olecranon bursae bilaterally are characteristic of tophaceous gout.
- *Rheumatoid nodules:* The absence of typical rheumatoid arthropathic changes and the dense olecranon bursal deposits of uric acid crystals exclude this diagnosis.
- *Tumoral calcinosis:* The clinical presentation is not consistent with this diagnosis.

■ Essential Facts

- In the group of diseases collectively termed gout, arthritis results from a disturbance of urate metabolism in which monosodium urate crystals are deposited in the joints and soft tissues.
- The diagnosis of gout is based on the identification of uric acid crystals in joints, tissues, or body fluids.
- In tophaceous gout, urate, protein matrix, inflammatory cells, and foreign body giant cells are deposited in the soft tissues.
- These deposits tend to occur around the olecranon bursae and the cartilage of the ear, nose, and menisci.
- Tophaceous gout occurs in < 10% of patients with gout and is seen more frequently in men in the fifth to seventh decades of life.
- Tophaceous deposits in the absence of arthritis may occasionally be the initial manifestation of gout.

✔ Pearls & ✘ Pitfalls

- ✔ Gouty tophi typically show isointense magnetic resonance (MR) imaging signal on T1-weighted images and heterogeneous low to intermediate MR imaging signal intensity on T2-weighted images. Adjacent bony overgrowth from tophaceous inflammatory changes is common.
- ✘ Calcified tophaceous deposits may erode bone, mimicking a focal sclerotic or chondroid lesion of bone.

Case 73

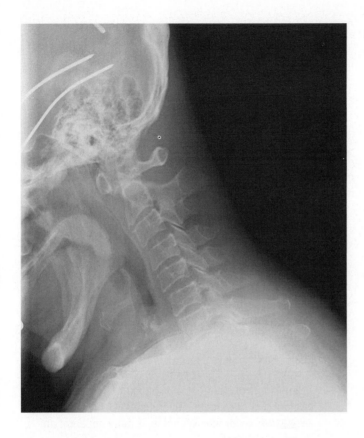

■ Clinical Presentation

··

The patient is a 63-year-old woman with a history of rheumatoid arthritis (RA).

■ Imaging Findings

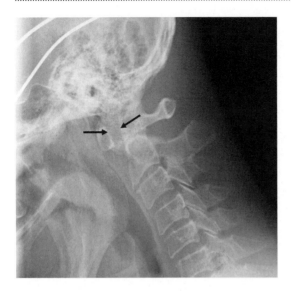

A lateral flexion view of the cervical spine shows widening of the predental space (*arrows*). The prevertebral soft tissues are normal.

■ Differential Diagnosis

- *Atlantoaxial subluxation:* Abnormal widening of the predental space is consistent with atlantoaxial subluxation.

■ Essential Facts

- Atlantoaxial subluxation results from a deficiency of the transverse ligament, which allows the dens to move posteriorly and superiorly relative to the atlas.
- Enlargement of the predental space, which should be 3 mm in adults, points to injury of this ligament.
- RA accounts for the majority of cases of atlantoaxial subluxation.
- This type of involvement of the cervical spine is seen in up to 60% of patients with RA.
- These patients are also at risk for spontaneous fracture of the dens and medullary compression.
- Many patients may be asymptomatic despite remarkable subluxation.
- The treatment for patients with instability is fusion.

✔ Pearls & ✗ Pitfalls

- ✔ Other causes of atlantoaxial subluxation include trauma, calcium pyrophosphate dihydrate (CPPD) arthropathy, and Downs syndrome. Widening is more apparent on flexion radiographs.
- ✗ The predental space in the pediatric cervical spine may appear falsely widened; the normal measurement ranges up to 5 mm.

Case 74

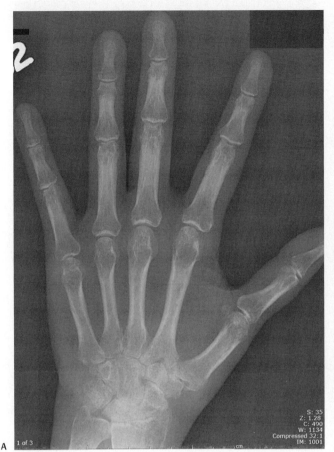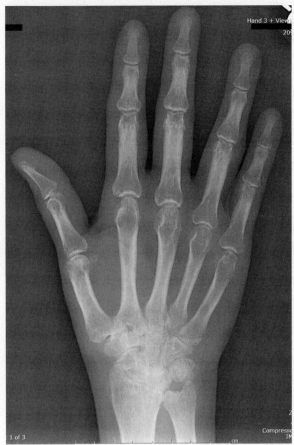

▪ Clinical Presentation

The patient is a 50-year-old woman with polyarthralgia.

■ Imaging Findings

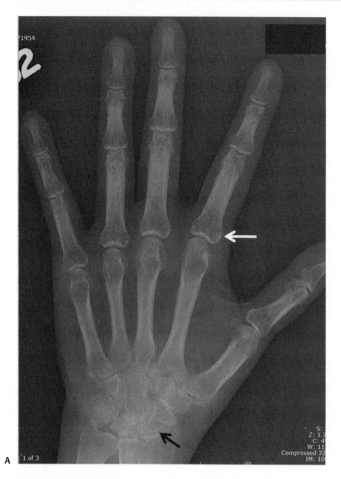
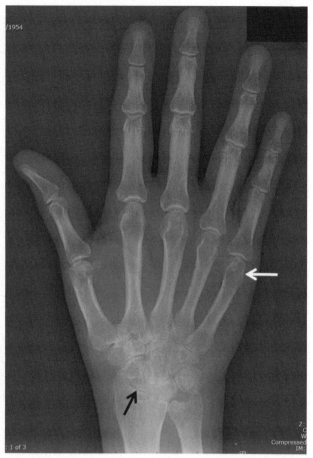

(A,B) Frontal radiographs of the hands show bilateral periarticular osteopenia (*white arrows*) and joint space loss across the wrist joints (*black arrows*) with the absence of osteophytes.

■ Differential Diagnosis

- ***Rheumatoid arthritis (RA):*** The female gender, symmetric distribution with periarticular osteopenia, and pancompartmental wrist joint space loss are characteristic of RA.
- *Osteoarthritis:* Symmetric periarticular osteopenia and diffuse wrist joint space loss without osteophytes is not consistent with osteoarthritis.
- *Psoriatic arthritis:* The symmetry and distribution of the findings and the absence of periostitis are not representative of psoriatic arthritis.

■ Essential Facts

- RA is a chronic systemic polyarticular disease that predominantly involves the synovial tissues and joints in a symmetric fashion.
- Circulating rheumatoid factor interacts with the synovial membranes, eliciting inflammatory changes responsible for the arthropathic changes of periarticular erosions, subluxations, joint space loss, osteopenia, and soft-tissue swelling.

- RA affects 0.5% to 1.0% of the global population, with women affected more frequently than men.
- Patients are typically 30 to 60 years of age.
- Symmetric involvement of the hands and wrists is common.
- Pancompartmental wrist joint space loss is related to synovitis and may be seen in the absence of digit involvement.
- Ulnar styloid erosions and metacarpophalangeal (MCP) and proximal interphalangeal (PIP) joint erosions with joint space loss are typical.

✔ Pearls & ✗ Pitfalls

- ✔ The second and third MCP joints and the third PIP joints may exhibit the earliest findings in RA.
- ✗ Gout and lupus arthropathy may appear similar to RA in the hand and wrist.

Case 75

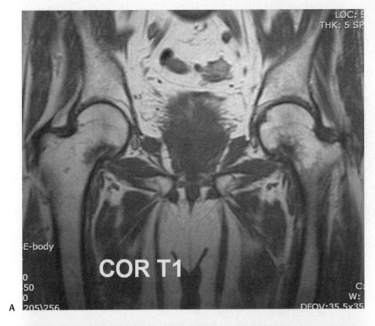

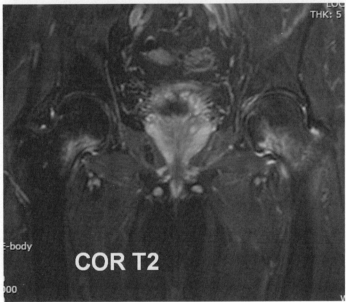

A

B

▨ Clinical Presentation

A 66-year-old man presents with bilateral atraumatic hip pain, osteopenia, and a history of chronic steroid use.

■ Imaging Findings

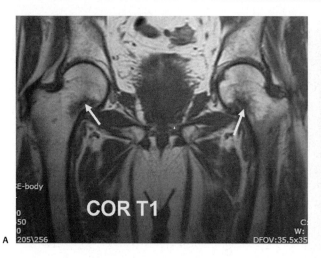
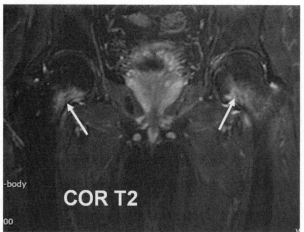

(A,B) Coronal magnetic resonance (MR) images through the hips show decreased T1 signal intensity and increased T2 signal intensity interrupting the normal corticomedullary junction along the inferior surface of each femoral neck (*arrows*).

■ Differential Diagnosis

- ***Insufficiency fractures:*** The history of steroid use, osteopenia, and localized edematous marrow changes in the femoral necks are representative of this diagnosis.
- *Avascular necrosis:* The location and pattern of the MR signal abnormality do not fit this diagnosis.
- *Osteomyelitis:* The history and localized corticomedullary MR findings argue against this diagnosis.

■ Essential Facts

- Insufficiency fractures are nonacute microfractures related to repetitive microtrauma.
- The underlying bone is typically osteoporotic.
- This process is generally seen in elderly patients and is acquired as a result of normal loading of the skeleton during activities of daily living.
- The femoral neck is one of the most common sites of insufficiency fractures.
- Radiographic findings of irregular sclerosis are most typical.
- If untreated, these injuries may progress to a complete fracture.

✔ Pearls & ✗ Pitfalls

- ✔ In the femoral neck, insufficiency fractures favor the subcapital region.
- ✗ Radiographic findings are often normal in the early stages of this injury.

Case 76

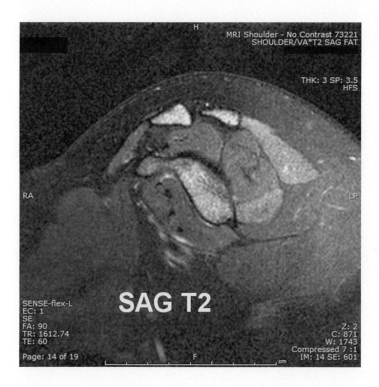

Clinical Presentation

A 19-year-old woman presents with chronic shoulder weakness and no history of trauma.

■ Imaging Findings

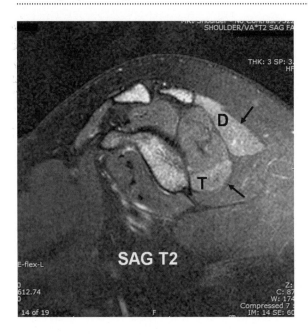

Mild edema (*arrows*) is present in the teres minor (*T*) and deltoid (*D*) muscles on oblique sagittal T2-weighted magnetic resonance (MR) images with fat suppression.

■ Differential Diagnosis

- ***Quadrilateral space syndrome:*** MR images revealing geographic denervation edema and/or fatty atrophy isolated to the teres minor and deltoid muscles in the absence of rotator cuff tendon pathology are diagnostic of quadrilateral space syndrome.
- *Suprascapular notch entrapment neuropathy*: This pattern of atrophy and/or edema typically involves the supraspinatus and infraspinatus muscles.
- *Spinoglenoid notch entrapment neuropathy*: This pattern of atrophy and/or edema typically involves the infraspinatus muscle.

■ Essential Facts

- Quadrilateral space syndrome is a clinical syndrome resulting from compression of the axillary nerve and posterior circumflex humeral artery in the quadrilateral space.
- The quadrilateral space is an anatomic region in the upper arm bounded by the long head of the triceps muscle, the teres minor and teres major muscles, and the cortex of the humerus.
- The clinical manifestations include poorly localized shoulder pain, paresthesias in the affected extremity, and discrete point tenderness in the lateral aspect of the quadrilateral space.
- The syndrome manifests with focal denervation edema and eventual atrophy involving the teres minor muscle with or without involvement of portions of the deltoid muscle.

- Axillary nerve compression is typically from fibrous bands thought to be secondary to prior trauma with resultant scarring.
- Surgery is usually reserved for patients whose condition is refractory to aggressive physical therapy.

✔ Pearls & ✗ Pitfalls

- ✔ The majority of these patients have no definable mass within the quadrilateral space on imaging.
- ✗ Brachial neuritis (Parsonage–Turner syndrome) may mimic quadrilateral space syndrome on MR images.

Case 77

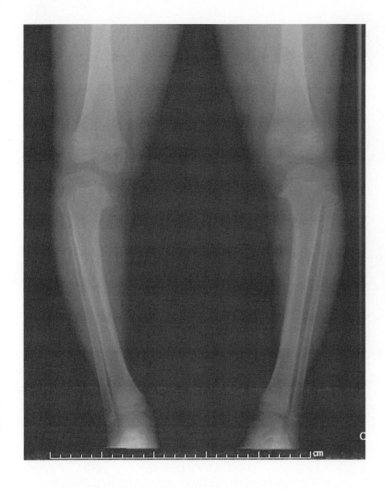

■ Clinical Presentation

The patient is a 4-year-old obese girl with bowlegs.

■ Imaging Findings

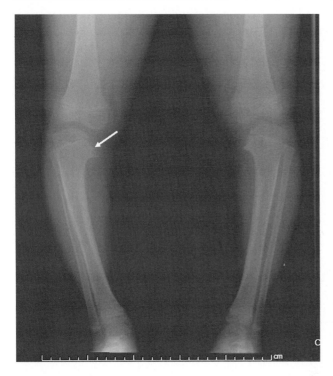

Frontal radiograph of the legs shows asymmetric depression and bony irregularity of the proximal tibial metaphyses, particularly on the right side (*arrow*), causing varus angulation. Abnormally tilted ankle joints are seen.

■ Differential Diagnosis

- ***Blount disease:*** Asymmetric tibia vara deformities associated with obesity and medial tibial metaphyseal depression associated with osseous irregularity/fragmentation are distinct features of Blount disease.
- *Achondroplasia*: These patients demonstrate metaphyseal flaring and cupping.
- *Physiologic bowing*: This process is typically symmetric without metaphyseal disturbances.

■ Essential Facts

- Blount disease, or tibia vara, is a common condition believed to result from abnormal stress on the posteromedial proximal tibial physis, which suppresses growth.
- The growth at the epiphysis becomes asymmetric, leading to the typical varus angulation.
- This process is usually unilateral or asymmetric.
- Predisposing factors for this disease are early walking, obesity, and African American descent.
- The physis may be widened medially because of arrested growth or laterally because of traction injury.

✔ Pearls & ✘ Pitfalls

- ✔ The medial tibial epiphyses are commonly deficient. Severe cases may show lateral tibial subluxation.
- ✘ Mild depression of the proximal tibial metaphyses posteromedially can occur with normal physiologic bowing.

Case 78

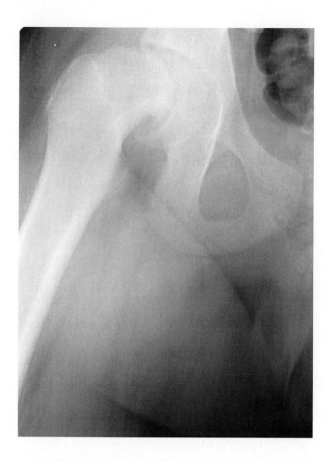

■ Clinical Presentation

The patient is a 14-year-old obese boy with chronic pain in the right hip.

■ Imaging Findings

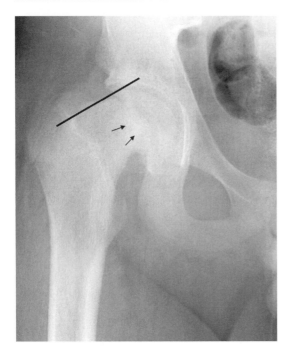

Radiograph of the right hip shows medial slippage of the epiphysis of the right femoral head, which is slightly flattened. The superior margin of the femoral neck (*line*) does not intersect the femoral head. Sclerotic remodeling along the metaphysis is present (*arrows*).

■ Differential Diagnosis

- ***Slipped capital femoral epiphysis (SCFE):*** Chronic hip pain and radiographic findings of medial slippage of the epiphysis of the femoral head in an obese adolescent boy are diagnostic of SCFE.
- *Salter–Harris type 1 fracture*: The chronic clinical and radiographic features and lack of major trauma do not allow this diagnosis.

■ Essential Facts

- SCFE is the most common abnormality of the hip in adolescence and a major cause of early osteoarthritis.
- It represents an atraumatic fracture through the physis.
- Males are affected more frequently than females, and the average age at presentation is 13 years.
- SCFE tends to affect overweight black males.
- Patients may present with weakness and/or pain in the thigh or knee.
- SCFE is bilateral in up to 37% of patients.
- Treatment typically consists of surgical pinning of the femoral epiphysis.

✔ Pearls & ✘ Pitfalls

- ✔ An early radiographic finding in SCFE is widening of the physis with surrounding demineralization.
- ✘ SCFE can be confused with a Salter–Harris type 1 fracture, which is less common and associated with major trauma.

Case 79

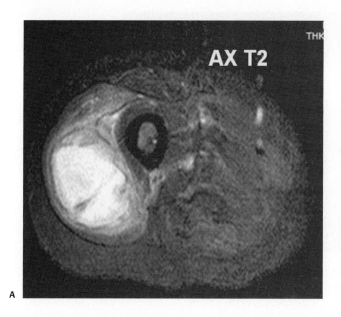

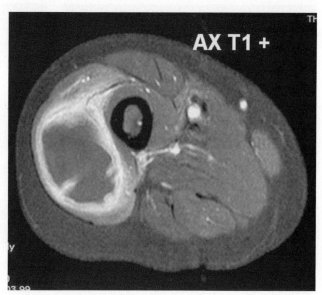

A

B

▪ Clinical Presentation

A 30-year-old patient who has AIDS presents with pain and redness in the right thigh.

■ Imaging Findings

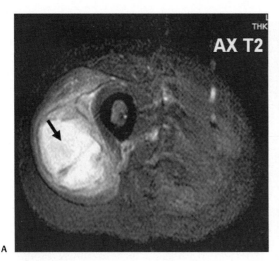
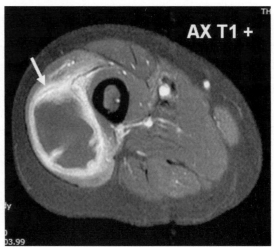

(A,B) Axial T2 weighted and contrast-enhanced, fat-suppressed T1-weighted magnetic resonance (MR) images demonstrate a mass involving the vastus lateralis muscle of the right midthigh. The post-contrast T1-weighted MR image shows thick rim enhancement (*white arrow*), and a central fluid signal (*black arrow*) is displayed on the T2-weighted image.

■ Differential Diagnosis

- ***Pyomyositis:*** This patient's history of AIDS and the redness and swelling combined with MR imaging findings of a rim-enhancing fluid collection are representative of pyomyositis.
- *Muscle necrosis*: T2 fluid signal with rim enhancement in solid muscle tissue is typical of this process.
- *Hematoma*: The MR imaging signal pattern of blood products is typically more heterogeneous and contains signal loss related to iron from hemoglobin by-products.

■ Essential Facts

- Pyomyositis is characterized by pyogenic inflammation of the muscle, most commonly due to *Staphylococcus aureus*.
- This is one of the most common musculoskeletal complications of AIDS. It is explained by the higher prevalence of intravenous drug abuse, rhabdomyolysis, and repetitive trauma in this population.
- These patients may present with fever and localized pain and swelling in the affected muscle.
- A palpable fluctuant mass can be present. Aspiration of the muscle reveals pus.
- Blood cultures are positive in only 5% of cases.
- The majority of patients require abscess drainage and surgical debridement.

✔ Pearls & ✘ Pitfalls

- ✔ Muscle necrosis with intramuscular gas may coexist with pyomyositis.
- ✘ Early MR imaging findings of pyomyositis are nonspecific and may appear as muscle edema.

Case 80

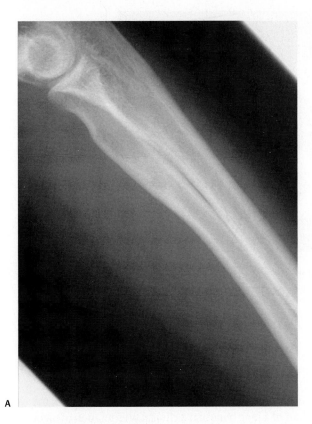

A

■ Clinical Presentation

The patient is an 11-year-old girl with nocturnal pain in her forearm.

Further Work-up

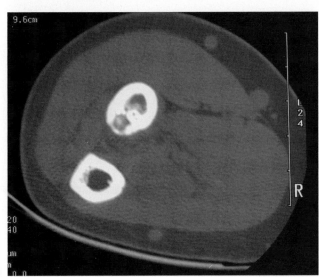

B

■ Imaging Findings

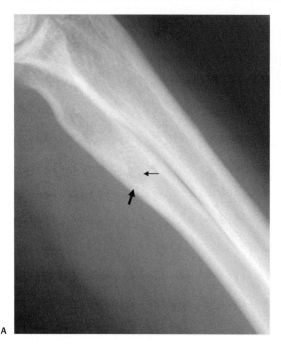

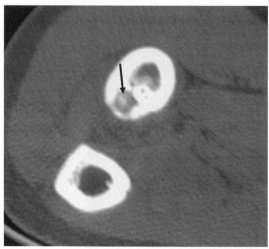

(A) Radiograph of the forearm display fusiform cortical thickening (*thick arrow*) encircling a faint lucency (*thin arrow*) in a proximal segment of the radial diaphysis. **(B)** Axial computed tomography (CT) through the proximal forearm shows an organized calcified nidus (*arrow*) embedded in the cortical thickening.

■ Differential Diagnosis

- *Osteoid osteoma*: Fusiform cortical thickening with a calcified nidus in a long bone accompanied by nocturnal pain is typical of osteoid osteoma.
- *Brodie's abscess*: The organized CT findings and clinical presentation are not characteristic of infection.
- *Stress fracture*: The clinical presentation, location, and nidus are not typical of a stress injury.

■ Essential Facts

- Osteoid osteomas are nonmalignant cortex-based neoplasms composed of osteoid. They account for ~12% of all benign skeletal lesions.
- This lesion is common in young males.
- Patients present with night pain that is relieved by salicylates.
- This neoplasm is most common in the tibial and femoral diaphyses.
- Patients can be successfully treated with radio-frequency thermal ablation.

✔ Pearls & ✘ Pitfalls

- ✔ Fusiform cortical thickening with a central nidus in the shaft of a long bone and a clinical presentation of night pain relieved by salicylates are diagnostic of osteoid osteoma.
- ✘ Not all osteoid osteomas have a classic presentation, and the imaging findings may overlap with those of Brodie's abscess.

Case 81

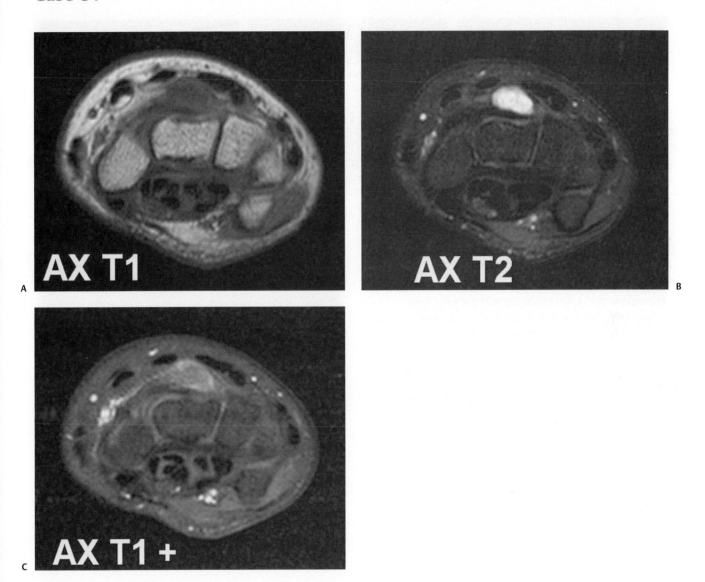

A AX T1

B AX T2

C AX T1 +

■ Clinical Presentation

A 24-year-old woman presents with a mass in the right wrist and normal radiographic findings.

■ Imaging Findings

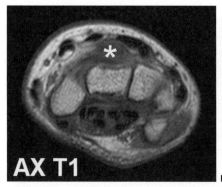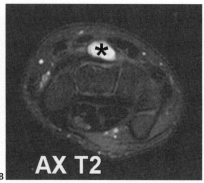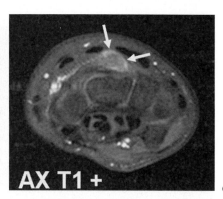

(A–C) Axial magnetic resonance (MR) images through the wrist show a focal fluid/cystic mass (*asterisk*) with wall enhancement (*arrows*) adhering to the soft tissues over the dorsum of the wrist.

■ Differential Diagnosis

- **Ganglion cyst:** A soft-tissue mass of the wrist with fluid/cystic MR signal characteristics demonstrating rim enhancement after the administration of gadolinium is characteristic of a ganglion cyst.
- *Tophaceous gout*: These lesions show marked heterogeneity on MR images.
- *Synovial sarcoma*: This is a solid lesion with aggressive growth characteristics.

■ Essential Facts

- Ganglion cysts are encapsulated foci of myxomatous degenerative tissue located adjacent to joints, ligaments, or tendons.
- The cyst is lined by fibrous tissue that enhances following the intravenous administration of gadolinium.
- Ganglion cysts should not be confused with synovial cysts, which are lined by synovium and contain synovial fluid.
- The origin of ganglion cysts is not uniformly agreed upon.
- However, a traumatic etiology is likely.
- Ganglion cysts of the dorsum of the wrist are most common and occur over the scapholunate ligament.
- Surgical resection is often required to prevent recurrence.

✔ Pearls & ✘ Pitfalls

- ✔ The most common soft-tissue mass around the wrist is a ganglion cyst.
- ✘ Small synovial cysts appear identical to ganglion cysts on MR images.

Case 82

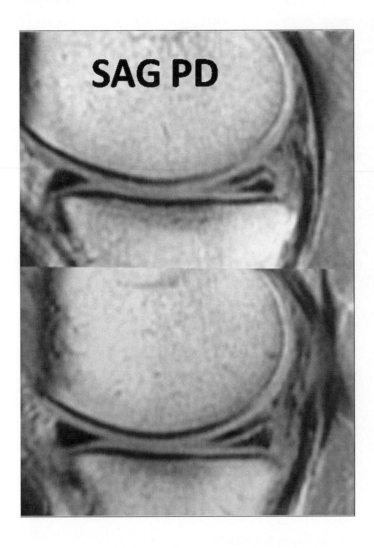

Clinical Presentation

A 50-year-old man presents with chronic knee pain.

■ Imaging Findings

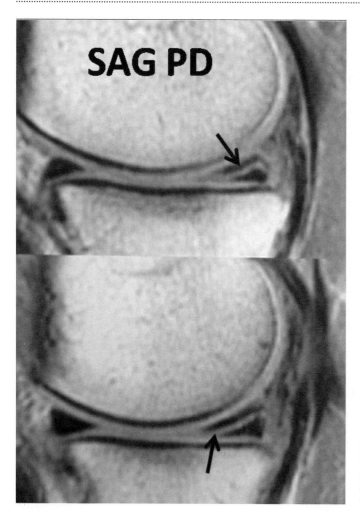

Sagittal proton density (PD) images through the posterior horn of the medial meniscus demonstrate increased signal (*arrows*) bisecting the posterior horn and extending to the tibial articular surface. The tear causes a cleavage plane between the cranial and caudal segments of this portion of the meniscus.

■ Differential Diagnosis

- *Horizontal cleavage meniscal tear:* Abnormally increased signal on proton density– and T2-weighted images that bisects the meniscus, dividing it into superior and inferior segments, and extends to an articular surface is representative of this type of meniscal tear.

■ Essential Facts

- Horizontal cleavage meniscal tears are parallel to the tibial plateau and divide the meniscus into upper and lower segments.
- To qualify as a meniscal tear, an area of abnormal signal must be seen within the meniscus on at least one image that extends to the articular surface of the meniscus.
- Degenerative joint disease usually produces these types of tears in the posterior half of the medial meniscus.
- As a result, these tears are more common in older patients.

✔ Pearls & ✗ Pitfalls

- ✔ Horizontal cleavage tears are the most common type of tear to be associated with a meniscal cyst. The posterior horn of the medial meniscus is the most common location for meniscal tears.
- ✗ A false-positive finding of a meniscal tear can occur with a healed meniscal tear or after surgical repair of a meniscal tear.

Case 83

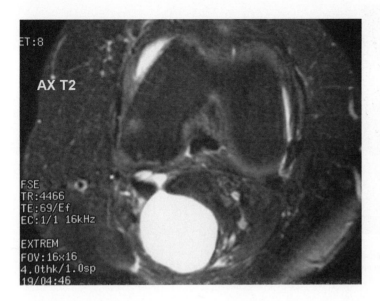

■ Clinical Presentation

A 50-year-old woman presents with a palpable mass in the medial popliteal fossa.

■ Imaging Findings

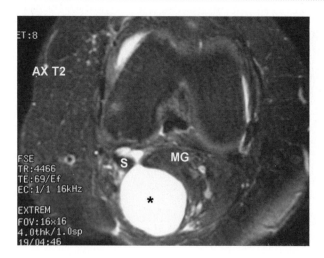

Axial T2-weighted magnetic resonance image shows a hyperintense fluid collection (*asterisk*) in the posteromedial knee, located between the medial gastrocnemius muscle (*MG*) and the semimembranosus tendon (*S*).

■ Differential Diagnosis

- **Baker's cyst:** A cyst interposed between the medial gastrocnemius muscle and semimembranosus tendon is diagnostic.
- *Myxoid liposarcoma*: The lack of internal fatty septa argues against this diagnosis. Additionally, post-contrast imaging (not provided) will show internal areas of enhancement.
- *Meniscal cyst*: This location is not typical of the plane of dissection of a meniscal cyst.

■ Essential Facts

- A Baker's cyst or popliteal cyst is the most common type of cyst located about the knee.
- This is a fluid-filled semimembranosus tendon–medial gastrocnemius bursa located in the medial popliteal region of the knee.
- It results from any condition that causes a joint effusion.
- The weakness of the posterior joint capsule allows the cyst to be connected to the posterior knee joint. The prevalence increases with age and is significantly higher in patients older than 50 years. A strong association with an internal derangement of the knee is noted. These cysts may rupture and dissect into adjacent soft tissues, causing symptoms simulating those of deep venous thrombosis.

✔ Pearls & ✘ Pitfalls

- ✔ Tears of the posterior horn of the medial meniscus commonly coexist with Baker's cysts.
- ✘ Internal hemorrhage or synovial proliferation may obscure detection of these cysts.

Case 84

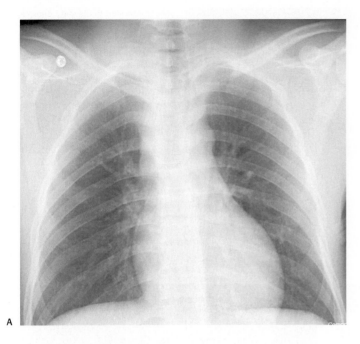

A

■ Clinical Presentation

A 20-year-old man presents with chest trauma after a motor vehicle crash.

Further Work-up

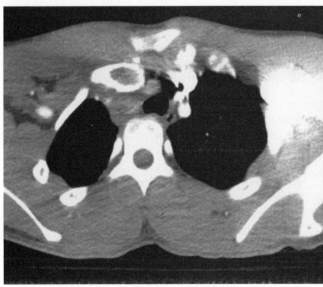

B

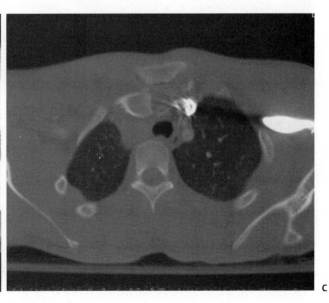

C

■ Imaging Findings

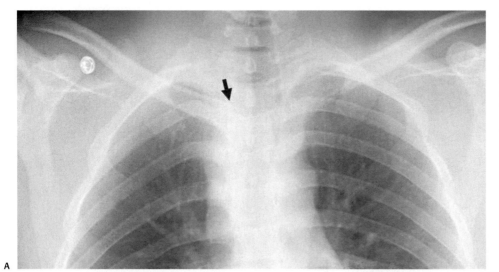

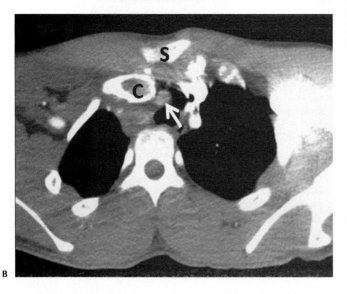

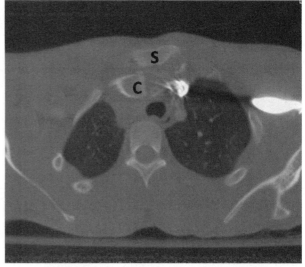

(A) Frontal view of the chest demonstrates offset of the sternoclavicular joints, with the right clavicular head directed caudally (*arrow*). **(B,C)** Axial computed tomographic (CT) scans demonstrate a posterior dislocation of the right clavicular head (*C*) relative to the sternum (*S*). The clavicular head medially displaces a branch vessel (*arrow*) of the aortic arch.

■ Differential Diagnosis

- **Posterior sternoclavicular joint dislocation:** The asymmetry of the sternoclavicular joints on radiography combined with the history raises suspicion for this dislocation. Contrast-enhanced CT confirms the dislocation and vascular impingement by the clavicular head.

■ Essential Facts

- Sternoclavicular joint dislocations account for 1% to 3% of all types of dislocations.
- Sternoclavicular dislocations may be anterior or posterior.
- Anterior sternoclavicular dislocations are more common and typically are evident on clinical examination by palpation and inspection.
- Posterior dislocations are more serious.
- The displaced clavicle can impinge on the underlying mediastinal vessels and nerves, esophagus, and trachea.

- A posterior dislocation can result directly from trauma to the anterior chest wall or indirectly from force applied to the ipsilateral posterior shoulder, which drives the lateral end of the clavicle anteriorly and causes the medial end of the clavicle to dislocate posteriorly.
- When this entity is suspected clinically, CT with the intravenous administration of contrast material can be used to confirm the diagnosis.
- Open reduction by an orthopedic surgeon with the assistance of a cardiothoracic surgeon may be required to treat this injury safely.

✔ Pearls & ✗ Pitfalls

✔ Contrast-enhanced CT of the chest is the gold standard for evaluating this injury, which is often occult on clinical examination.

✗ Posterior sternoclavicular dislocations may be subtle or not visualized at all on conventional radiography.

Case 85

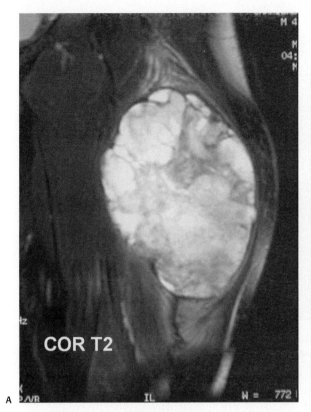

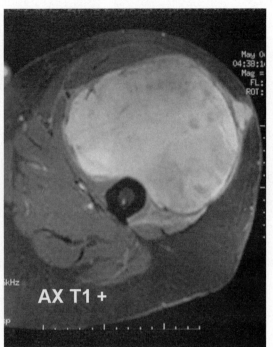

A

B

■ Clinical Presentation

A 40-year-old man presents with an enlarging mass in the left thigh.

■ Imaging Findings

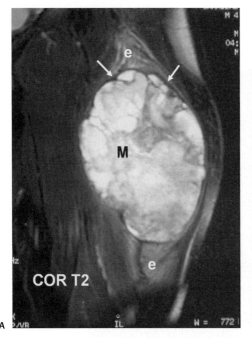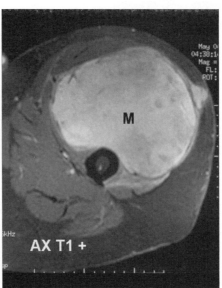

(A,B) Magnetic resonance (MR) images through the left thigh show a large, solid mass (*M*) infiltrating the quadriceps musculature. Heterogeneous T2 signal increase is present, with solid enhancement and surrounding muscle edema (*e*). A low-signal capsule (*arrows*) encircles the mass.

■ Differential Diagnosis

- ***Malignant fibrous histiocytoma (MFH):*** The patient's age, the intramuscular location in a lower extremity, and solid, heterogeneous characteristics on MR images point to this malignancy.
- *Hematoma*: The MR image characteristics, particularly the solid nature of the lesion and lack of artifact from blood products, exclude this diagnosis.
- *Liposarcoma*: This diagnosis is unlikely, but not impossible, given the absence of fat signal.

■ Essential Facts

- MFH is the most common soft-tissue sarcoma in adults, showing a male predilection. The peak incidence is in the 5th and 6th decades.
- The lower extremity is involved in 50% of cases.
- Two thirds of these lesions have a deep intramuscular location.
- The typical patient presents with a painless, enlarging soft-tissue mass.
- Radiographs of MFH typically reveal an indeterminate soft-tissue mass with mineralization in 5 to 20% of cases.
- Deep intramuscular lesions may cause extrinsic erosion of adjacent long bones.
- MR images will show a large, lobulated, well-circumscribed mass with intermediate signal intensity on T1-weighted images and high signal intensity on T2-weighted images.

- The lesions are usually heterogeneous because of the varied cellularity and cell types. Non-necrotic areas of the tumor usually demonstrate marked enhancement.
- Lesions may display a relatively well-defined margin reflecting a surrounding pseudocapsule.
- Spontaneous hemorrhage within this tumor is not uncommon, and a diagnosis of MFH should be considered in any adult presenting with a spontaneous hematoma.

✔ Pearls & ✘ Pitfalls

✔ A knowledge of the prevalence of soft-tissue tumors according to location and age, along with an appropriate clinical history and radiologic features, can be used to establish this diagnosis with a reasonable degree of certainty.

✘ One cannot differentiate reliably between benign and malignant soft-tissue lesions with radiologic imaging alone.

Case 86

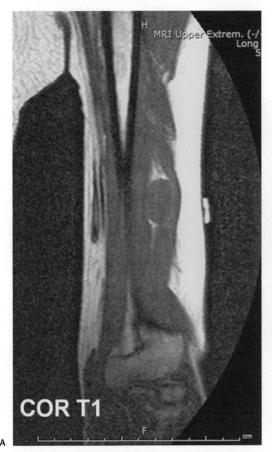

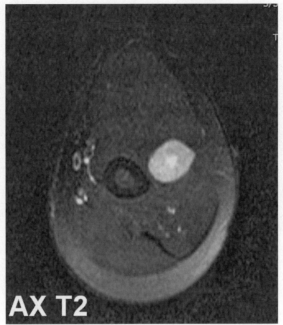

■ Clinical Presentation

A 38-year-old man has a history of a palpable mass in the left arm with paresthesias.

■ Imaging Findings

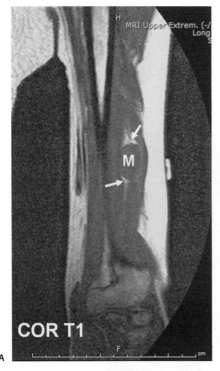

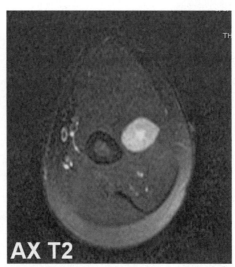

(A,B) Coronal T1-weighted magnetic resonance (MR) image of the arm shows a fusiform mass (*M*) containing homogeneous and isointense signal intensity relative to skeletal muscle. This lesion is located along the course of the radial nerve. A subtle rind of fat is seen at the margins of the mass (*arrows*). Axial T2-weighted MR image shows a heterogeneous signal increase within the lesion, particularly in the center.

■ Differential Diagnosis

- **Nerve sheath tumor:** A history of paresthesias and a fusiform mass with isointense T1 signal that runs parallel to the radial nerve and is located within fat are characteristic of a nerve sheath tumor.

■ Essential Facts

- Peripheral nerve sheath tumors include schwannomas and neurofibromas.
- Schwannomas are slightly less common than neurofibromas.
- Patients typically present with paresthesias and a slowly enlarging mass that is painless on palpation.
- Schwannomas arise from the epineurium and are characteristically eccentric with respect to the affected nerve, which is displaced to the periphery of the mass.
- The fusiform morphology relates to the longitudinal growth pattern.
- Neurofibromas arise from the nerve fascicle and are centrally located.
- When large nerves are affected, the relationship between the native nerve and the mass may make it possible to distinguish between these two lesions.

- A peripheral nerve sheath tumor should be suspected when a mass is located in the region of a major nerve and the nerve is depicted entering or exiting the mass.
- The mass effect causes the surrounding fat to separate, giving rise to the "split-fat" sign seen on MR images.
- The target sign has been described on T2-weighted MR images of neurogenic tumors and is characterized by low signal intensity centrally and high signal intensity peripherally. These findings correspond to the central fibrous components and peripheral myxomatous elements seen at pathologic analysis.
- The target sign is seen more frequently in neurofibromas, although it may also be apparent in schwannomas.

✔ Pearls & ✘ Pitfalls

- ✔ MR imaging characteristics of nerve sheath tumors include the split-fat sign and the target sign.
- ✘ It can be difficult to differentiate between schwannomas and neurofibromas when the tumors are associated with small nerves.

Case 87

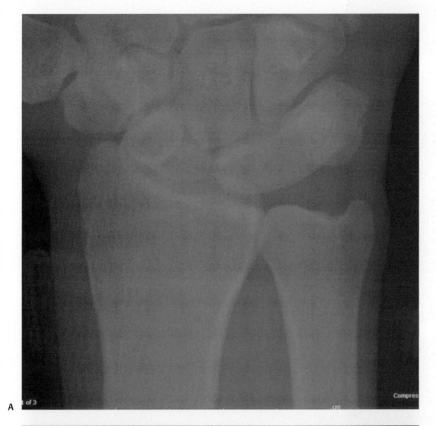

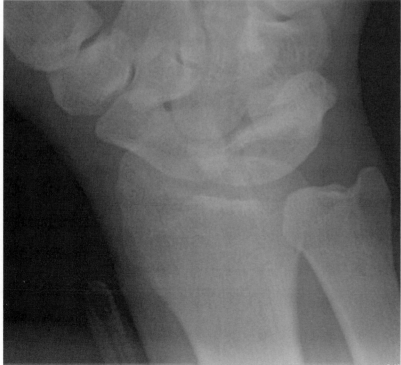

■ Clinical Presentation

A 30-year-old man presents with wrist pain after a fall.

■ Imaging Findings

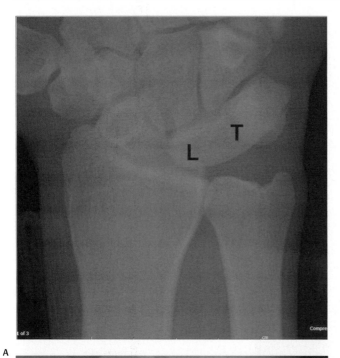

A

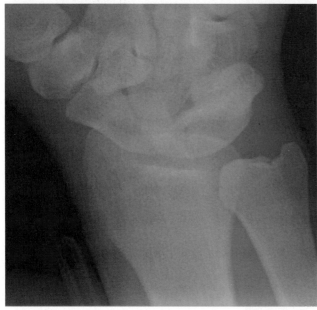

B

(A,B) Radiographs of the wrist show osseous fusion between the lunate (*L*) and triquetrum (*T*). No acute bony abnormality is seen.

■ Differential Diagnosis

- **Lunotriquetral coalition:** The absence of an articulation between the lunate and triquetrum on multiple radiographic projections is diagnostic of carpal coalition.

■ Essential Facts

- Carpal coalition in isolation is a fairly common variant.
- It is most commonly seen between the lunate and triquetrum and is related to segmentation failure of the carpal bones.
- Fusions are bilateral in > 50% of cases.

- Coalitions are usually discovered incidentally. They are painless and not associated with functional instability.
- Partial coalitions may present with wrist pain.
- Extensive carpal coalitions can be seen with congenital malformation syndromes.

✔ Pearls & ✘ Pitfalls

- ✔ Isolated carpal coalitions involve bony structures in the same carpal row.
- ✘ Scapholunate widening may be seen with this condition in the absence of ligamentous disruption.

Case 88

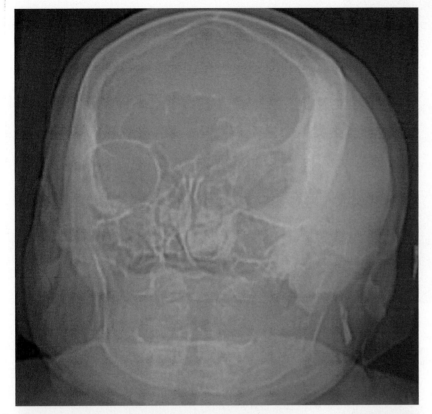

A

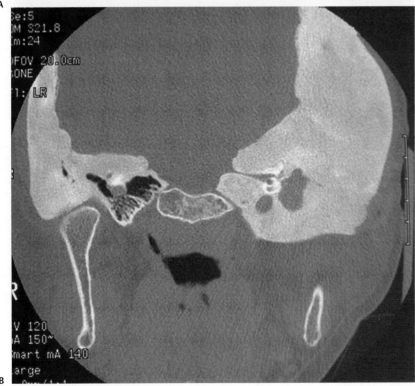

B

■ Clinical Presentation

The patient is a 46-year-old man with facial deformity.

■ Imaging Findings

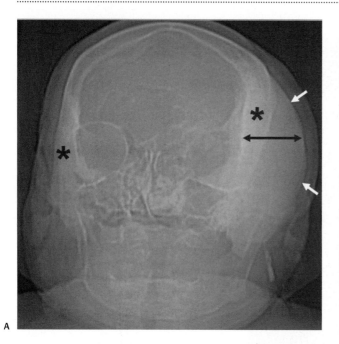

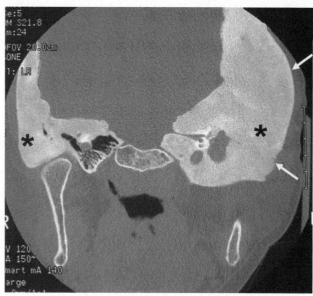

A

B

(A) Frontal radiograph of the skull demonstrates a ground glass appearance of the diploic space (*asterisks*), which is markedly expanded (*double-headed arrow*). This expansion causes an outward convex deformation of the outer table (*arrows*). These findings are more notable on the left. **(B)** Primarily outward calvarial expansion is seen on a coronal computed tomographic (CT) scan (*arrows*), with a hazy/smoky appearance of the diploic space (*asterisks*).

■ Differential Diagnosis

- **Fibrous dysplasia (FD):** Ground glass replacement/expansion of the craniofacial diploic space with convex deformity of the outer table of the skull is pathognomonic for FD.
- *Paget's disease*: The concomitant involvement of the cranial and facial bones with ground glass matrix replacement is not typical of Paget's disease.
- *Metastasis*: The organized geographic pattern of craniofacial involvement with a ground glass matrix is not consistent with metastasis.

■ Essential Facts

- FD is a bone disorder characterized by overgrowth of the marrow with fibro-osseous tissue.
- Monostotic and polyostotic variants are seen.
- The craniofacial bones are involved in 20% of cases of monostotic FD and in 50% of cases of polyostotic FD.
- Involvement of the frontal, sphenoid, maxillary, and ethmoid regions is typical.
- Patients may present with neurologic symptoms related to foraminal encroachment resulting from osseous expansion.
- CT is valuable for evaluating the extent of osseous involvement in the skull. This disease typically becomes quiescent at puberty.

✔ Pearls & ✘ Pitfalls

- ✔ The osseous expansion of the skull is frequently in an outward direction, such that the outer table of the skull is convex.
- ✘ Early craniofacial changes of FD are not detectable on radiography.

Case 89

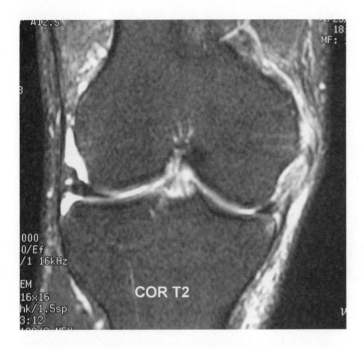

■ Clinical Presentation

After trauma, a patient presents with medial joint line tenderness and a possible meniscal tear.

■ Imaging Findings

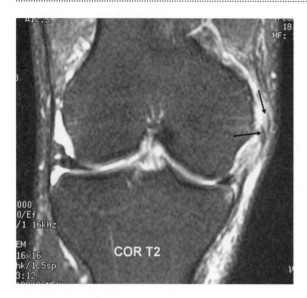

Coronal T2-weighted magnetic resonance (MR) image reveals complete disruption of the proximal medial collateral ligament (MCL: *arrows*) with fluid surrounding the medial ligamentous structures of the knee.

■ Differential Diagnosis

• ***Medial collateral ligament tear:*** Complete disruption of the normally low-signal fibers of the MCL with intervening increased T2 signal is characteristic of this injury.

■ Essential Facts

• The MCL is an important stabilizer of the medial portion of the knee. Injuries to this ligament are caused by a blow to the lateral aspect of the knee or proximal tibia.
• MCL tears are classified according to the degree of injury. In a first-degree tear, the fibers are intact but stretched; a third-degree tear is complete fiber disruption.
• The most common injuries associated with MCL tears are anterior cruciate ligament tears, medial meniscal tears, meniscocapsular separations, and medial retinaculum disruption.

✔ Pearls & ✘ Pitfalls

✔ MCL disruption is best evaluated on coronal MR images. Tears of the MCL most commonly occur at the femoral origin.
✘ Nontraumatic inflammatory processes can cause fluid to form around the MCL, mimicking a tear.

Case 90

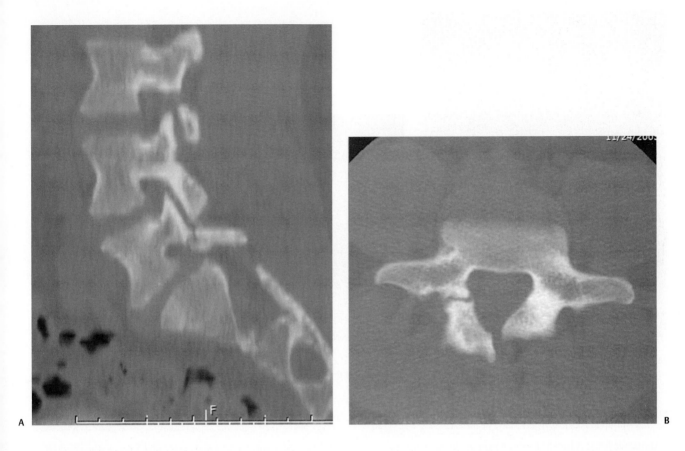

A   B

■ Clinical Presentation

A 17-year-old high school football player presents with chronic low back pain.

■ Imaging Findings

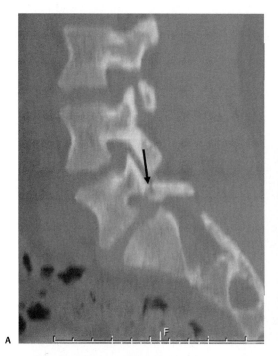
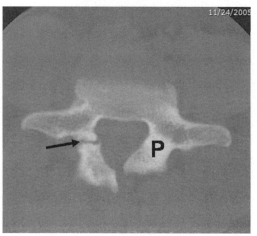

A   B

(A,B) Sagittal and axial computed tomographic scans demonstrate a right-sided defect of the L5 pars interarticularis with irregular marginal sclerosis (*arrows*). Sclerotic remodeling and enlargement of the contralateral pedicle (*P*) are seen.

■ Differential Diagnosis

• **Spondylolysis:** A lucent defect through the pars interarticularis that is surrounded by sclerosis with compensatory sclerosis and enlargement of the contralateral pedicle is diagnostic of this condition.

■ Essential Facts

• Spondylolysis is a stress fracture of the pars interarticularis related to overuse.
• It is associated with repetitive hyperextension of the spine and is much more common in children and adolescents than in adults.
• Gymnastics, ballet, and football are particularly common associated activities.
• Acute or chronic pain, typically aggravated during extension, is the most frequent presenting complaint.
• Spondylolysis is rare at levels above the lumbar spine.
• Bilateral spondylolysis may be complicated by spondylolisthesis, which is anterior subluxation of the body of the involved vertebra.
• Lateral lumbar spinal radiographs are often useful and may demonstrate a radiolucency crossing the pars interarticularis. Sclerosis may be evident as a result of healing at the fracture site.

✔ Pearls & ✗ Pitfalls

✔ The L4-L5 and L5-S1 levels are most frequently affected by this process.
✗ The diagnosis of spondylolysis by magnetic resonance imaging can be quite difficult and is generally not recommended.

Case 91

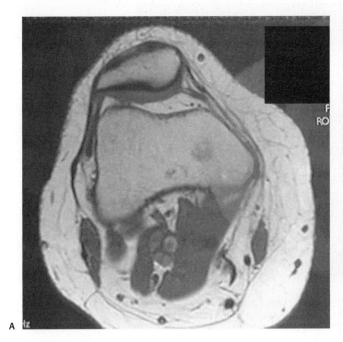 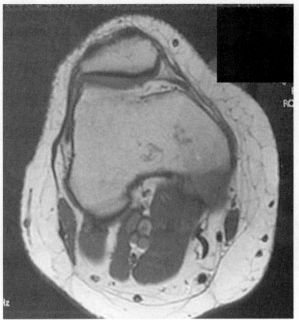

A

B

■ Clinical Presentation

A 35-year-old woman presents with intermittent claudication of the calf.

■ Imaging Findings

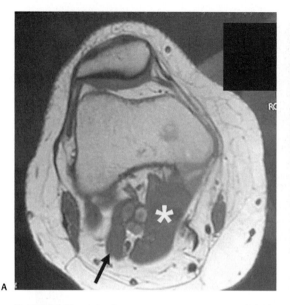 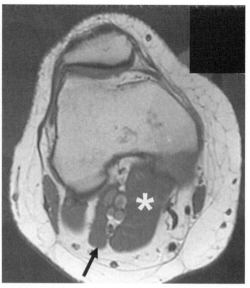

(A,B) Axial T1-weighted magnetic resonance images of the knee demonstrate an accessory slip of the medial head of the gastrocnemius (*arrows*) arising from the posterior aspect of the distal femur. This slip forms a lateral sling around the popliteal vessels. A normal medial head of the gastrocnemius (*asterisk*) is situated medial to the popliteal vessels.

■ Differential Diagnosis

- **Popliteal artery entrapment:** An accessory slip of the medial head of the gastrocnemius forming a lateral sling around the popliteal artery in a patient with claudication of the calf is diagnostic of this vascular entrapment.

■ Essential Facts

- Popliteal artery entrapment is a developmental abnormality resulting from an abnormal relationship of the popliteal artery to the gastrocnemius muscle or, rarely, an anomalous fibrous band of the popliteus muscle.
- The abnormal position of the muscle causes the artery to deviate.
- Occlusion of the popliteal artery occurs on active plantar flexion or passive dorsiflexion of the ankle.
- Four muscular–vascular anatomic variants have been described.
- These patients are typically younger than 30 years of age and present with claudication of the calf and, rarely, ischemia due to thrombosis.
- Stress angiography is usually performed to confirm the diagnosis before surgery.
- If left untreated, entrapment may progress to permanent narrowing of the popliteal artery.
- Surgical release of the muscle or tendon is the ultimate treatment.

✔ Pearls & ✘ Pitfalls

- ✔ Bilateral popliteal artery involvement has been reported in up to 67% of presenting patients.
- ✘ A normally located artery may become entrapped by a hypertrophic gastrocnemius muscle.

Case 92

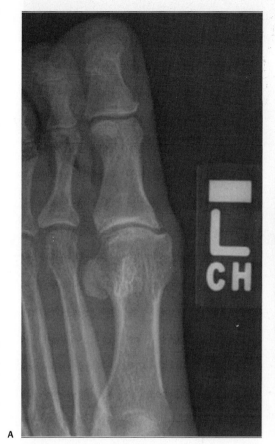

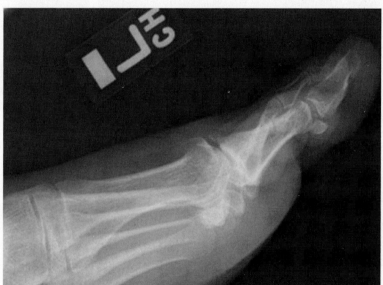

A

B

■ **Clinical Presentation**

A middle-aged woman presents with chronic pain in the left foot, decreased range of motion, and a palpable mass.

■ Imaging Findings

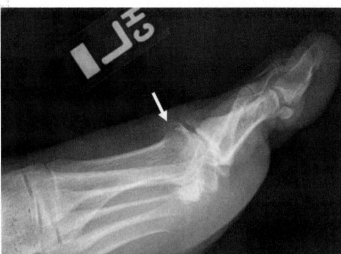

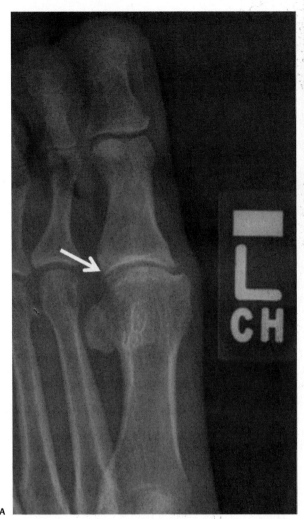

(A,B) Radiographs of the left forefoot demonstrate localized first metatarsophalangeal (MTP) joint space narrowing, subchondral sclerosis, and osteophyte formation (*arrows*). No erosions, subluxations, or osteopenia is seen.

■ Differential Diagnosis

- **Hallux rigidus:** The presence of dorsal osteophytes, bone sclerosis, and joint space loss predominantly in the first MTP joint of the forefoot in conjunction with the clinical history suggests this diagnosis.
- *Psoriatic arthritis*: The absence of erosions/periostitis and sparing of the interphalangeal joint exclude this diagnosis.
- *Rheumatoid arthritis*: The absence of erosive articular changes and osteopenia makes this an unlikely diagnosis.

■ Essential Facts

- Osteoarthrosis of the first MTP joint is termed *hallux rigidus.* This process is a consequence of damage to the articular cartilage resulting from repetitive microtrauma throughout the life process.
- It tends to involve specific synovial joints during specific decades of a person's life and depends in part on the patient's level of physical activity.

- The presence of osteophytes with bone sclerosis and the absence of inflammatory features such as erosions suggest this diagnosis.
- As the joint space narrows, the osteophytes may become larger. Involvement at the first MTP joint occurs twice as often in women.
- Progression of the disorder leads to painful restriction of dorsiflexion of the great toe and formation of a characteristic dorsal osteophyte that manifests clinically as a mass on examination.
- Hallux rigidus is common beginning in the 5th decade of life.

✔ Pearls & ✘ Pitfalls

- ✔ This process may be associated with a hallux valgus deformity and can be bilateral.
- ✘ Rarely, an inflammatory component of osteoarthrosis can occur about the foot, causing an appearance similar to that of an inflammatory/crystalline arthropathy.

Case 93

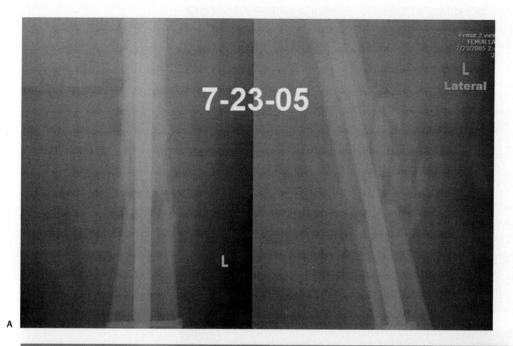

7-23-05

L

Lateral

L

A

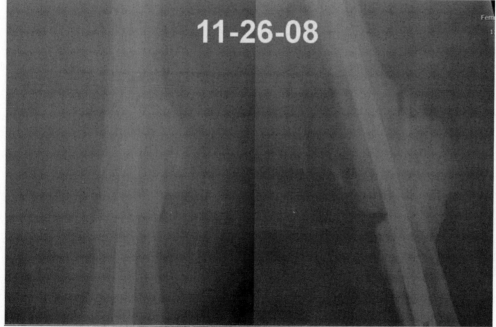

11-26-08

B

■ Clinical Presentation

The patient has a history of a fracture of the distal left femur with persistent pain and tenderness.

■ Imaging Findings

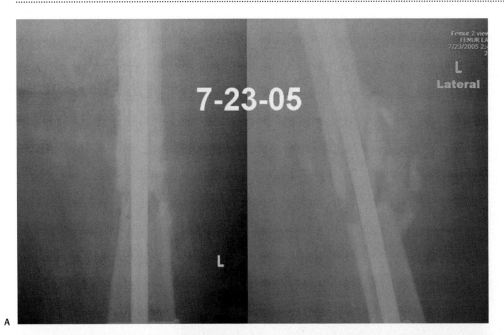

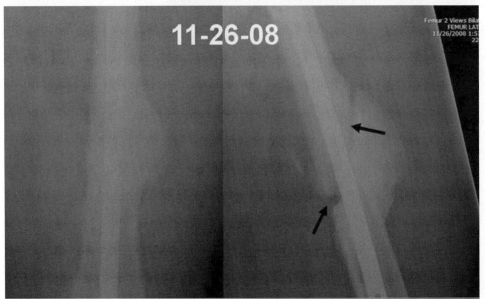

(A,B) Serial radiographs of the left femur performed > 3 years apart reveal a persistent comminuted fracture defect/pseudarthrosis (*arrows*) through the distal femoral diaphysis lined by hypertrophic bone. A superimposed intramedullary rod is in place.

■ Differential Diagnosis

- ***Hypertrophic non-union:*** The appearance of a fracture on radiographs > 9 months after an injury with surrounding hypertrophic bone represents this diagnosis.

■ Essential Facts

- Hypertrophic non-union is defined as failure of complete fracture healing on radiographs at 6 to 9 months following the date of injury.
- This process is typically related to abnormal immobilization across a fracture site.
- A pseudarthrosis is seen across the fracture bed which is outlined by bony hypertrophy.

- Non-union is most common in the long bones of adults, particularly the tibia and femur.
- Other important factors negatively affecting fracture healing include marked displacement of the fragments, infection, soft-tissue injury, poor blood supply, older age of the patient, and poor nutritional status.

✔ Pearls & ✘ Pitfalls

- ✔ Radiographic changes of hardware loosening may coexist with a hypertrophic non-union.
- ✘ Availability of prior radiographs may affect the ability to make this diagnosis.

Case 94

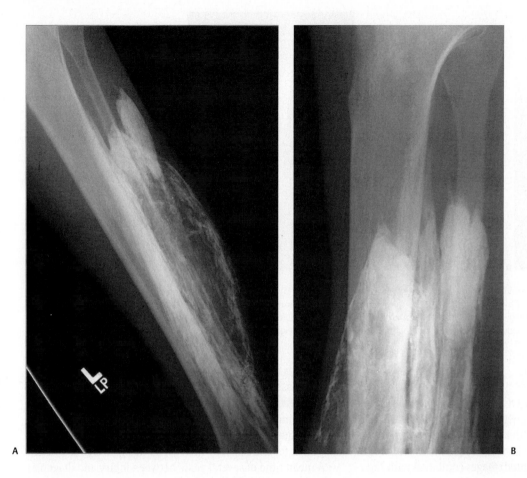

A
B

Clinical Presentation

A 60-year-old man presents with a several-year history of a slowly enlarging fluctuant mass in the left leg with a remote history of trauma.

Further Work-up

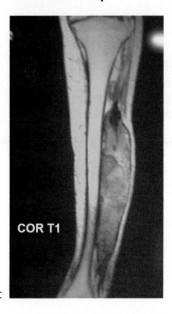

COR T1

C

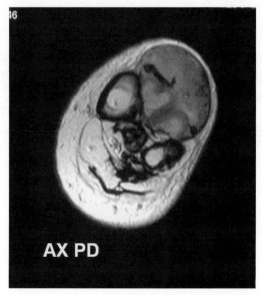

AX PD

D

■ Imaging Findings

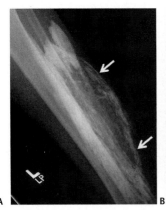
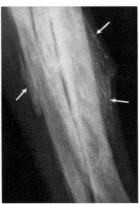
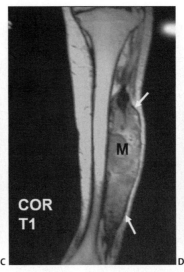
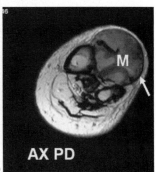

(A,B) Radiographs of the left tibia and fibula show a mineralized mass overlying the anterior compartment of the mid to distal leg. The calcifications are linear and platelike in morphology (*arrows*), with no bony matrix. **(C,D)** Magnetic resonance (MR) images show a fusiform, well-marginated soft-tissue mass (*M*) replacing the anterior compartment musculature. A peripheral rim of low signal intensity (*arrows*) surrounds this heterogeneous mass, which exhibits increased signal intensity on coronal T1- and axial proton density–weighted images.

■ Differential Diagnosis

- ***Calcific myonecrosis:*** A mass in the anterior compartment of the leg containing peripheral striated/linear, platelike calcifications is typical of this lesion. A complex cystic heterogeneous mass with increased signal intensity on T1- and proton density–weighted images combined with the history is also diagnostic of this process.
- *Myositis ossificans (MO):* The interval between the development of MO and the primary injury is short (weeks to months). This lesion has a trabecular pattern of calcification showing marrow signal on MR images. MO does not enlarge over time.
- *Hematoma*: Intramuscular hematomas do not replace muscle, and the calcifications tend to be more circumferential.

■ Essential Facts

- Calcific myonecrosis is a late sequela of trauma that occurs almost exclusively in the anterior compartment of the lower leg.
- It is thought that these lesions result from post-traumatic ischemia and cystic degeneration of the muscle.
- It is unique in that it involves and replaces an entire muscle or muscle compartment.
- Muscle replacement by a fusiform soft-tissue mass exhibiting peripheral linear, platelike calcifications and central liquefaction is typical.

- Patients may present with a painful, often expansive, calcified mass. The increasing size of the mass may be related to repeated intralesional hemorrhage, as suggested by the methemoglobin seen in some cases.
- Some authorities believe that proteinaceous debris accounts for the centrally increased MR signal characteristics.
- A mean time of several years between injury and diagnosis is common, given the insidious nature of this process.
- Because of the long delay between the primary injury and the clinical presentation of the mass, the history of trauma may be overlooked, causing confusion with other calcified soft-tissue masses.
- It is important to remember that these peripheral plaquelike calcifications do not represent bone formation.

✔ Pearls & ✘ Pitfalls

✔ Radiographically, the calcifications are parallel to the long axis of the compartment.
✘ Dystrophic calcifications, although different morphologically, may also occur as a result of abscess or diabetic myonecrosis.

Case 95

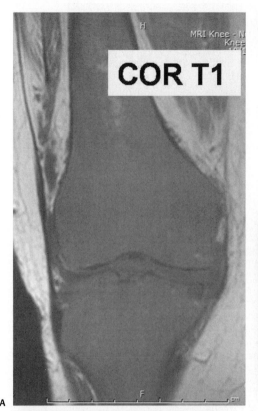

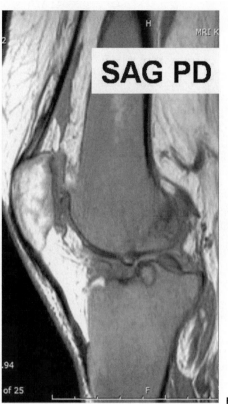

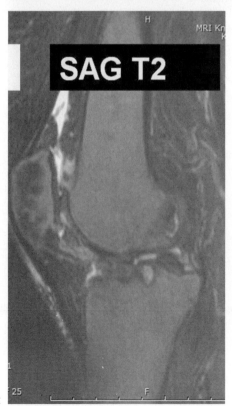

■ Clinical Presentation

A 63-year-old woman presents with fever, pain in the left leg, and leukocytosis.

■ Imaging Findings

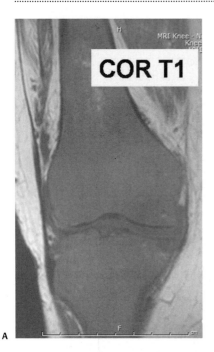
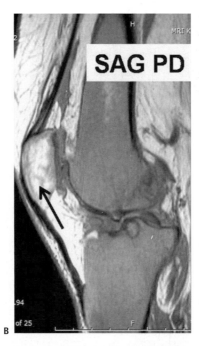
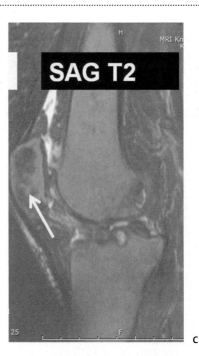

(A–C) Magnetic resonance (MR) images of the knee show replacement of the normal fatty marrow signal by diffuse low T1 signal and intermediate to increased proton density and T2 signal. The cortex is intact, without edema, a soft-tissue mass, or periostitis. Minimal normal fatty marrow signal remains in the patella (*arrows*).

■ Differential Diagnosis

- *Diffuse marrow infiltrative process:* Replacement of the normal fatty marrow signal by low T1 signal and intermediate to increased T2 and proton density signal is nonspecific yet signifies a systemic infiltrative process, which is chronic myelocytic leukemia in this case.

■ Essential Facts

- Yellow marrow is composed of 80% fat, 15% water, and 5% protein. These changes cause high T1 and low T2 (with fat suppression) MR signal.
- Hematopoetic or red marrow is composed of ~40% water, 40% fat, and 20% protein. Red marrow displays roughly opposite MR signal characteristics and predominates in the axial skeleton.
- Loss of normal marrow signal can be encountered in a multitude of diseases and normal marrow recovery states.
- Therapies to stimulate bone marrow following cancer treatment, anemia with hematopoetic replacement of fatty marrow, and neoplastic processes are a few of the causes.
- MR imaging findings of diffuse marrow infiltration by a systemic process are nonspecific.
- However, it is important to note that the normal marrow signal within the bony structures surrounding the knee in a healthy adult should resemble fat signal.
- Yellow marrow occupies most of the normal appendicular skeleton in an adult.

✔ Pearls & ✗ Pitfalls

✔ Metastatic disease typically destroys and replaces marrow elements, such as the osseous trabeculae, whereas marrow edema and hyperplastic red marrow do not.

✗ A significant proportion of patients with leukemia and myeloma may have normal marrow signal on MR imaging.

Case 96

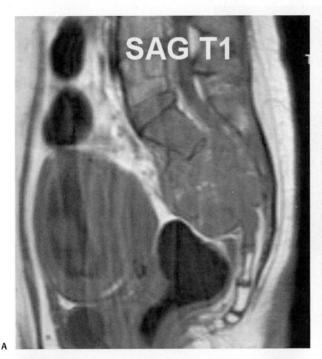

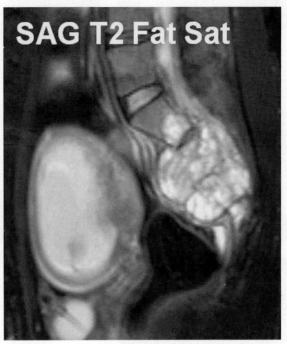

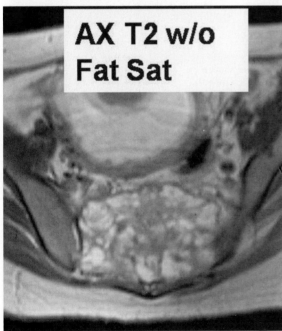

Clinical Presentation

The patient is a 19-year-old woman with a mass seen on prior obstetric ultrasonography.

■ Imaging Findings

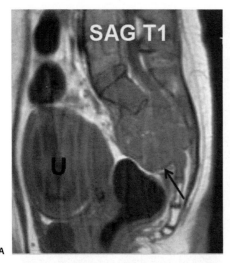

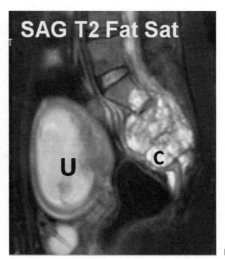

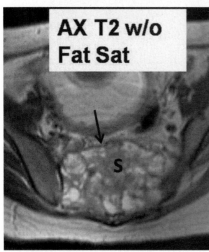

(A–C) Magnetic resonance (MR) images show a heterogeneous hyperintense, expansile, mixed cystic (*C*) and solid (*S*) mass deforming the sacrum. No internal calcifications or associated soft-tissue mass is grossly evident. A thin, low-signal rim (*arrows*) encloses the mass. A gravid uterus (*U*) is present.

■ Differential Diagnosis

- **Giant cell tumor (GCT):** An expansile, mixed cystic and solid complex sacral mass in this age group without a soft-tissue component or matrix mineralization is most consistent with a diagnosis of GCT.
- *Chordoma*: This midline sacral mass most commonly occurs in the 4th to 7th decades of life and exhibits internal calcifications accompanied by a large presacral soft-tissue component.
- *Aneurysmal bone cyst (ABC)*: This is a rare tumor within the sacrum that typically exhibits fluid–fluid levels.

■ Essential Facts

- GCT is the second most common primary sacral tumor after chordoma.
- It is most commonly seen in the 2nd to 4th decades of life.
- Spinal GCTs show a female predilection.
- These are locally aggressive and rarely may metastasize.
- The tumor is composed of giant cells, which are multi-nucleated macrophages.

- GCTs manifest as lytic, expansile, and destructive lesions that are often eccentrically located and contain a thin, sclerotic rim of bone.
- These are very vascular neoplasms that demonstrate significant enhancement on computed tomographic scans and MR images.
- They display intermediate signal intensity on both T1- and T2-weighted MR images and may contain areas of hemorrhage or necrosis.
- Their subchondral location in both long and flat bones may result in transarticular spread.
- In the sacrum, a GCT may show growth across the sacro-iliac joint to the ilium.

✔ Pearls & ✘ Pitfalls

- ✔ With respect to spinal involvement, the sacrum is the most common site for GCTs.
- ✘ Fluid–fluid levels may be present within a GCT, causing confusion with an ABC.

Case 97

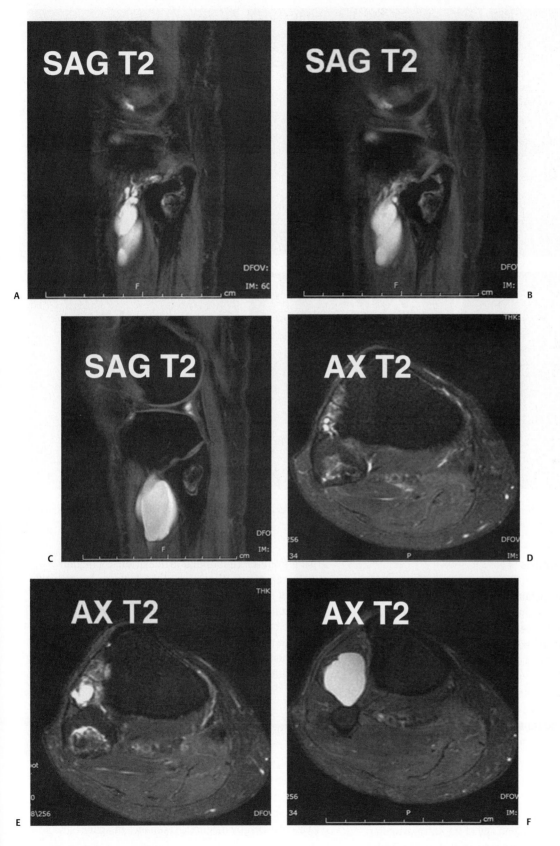

■ Clinical Presentation

The patient is a 74-year-old man with a palpable proximal leg mass, paresthesias, and footdrop.

■ Imaging Findings

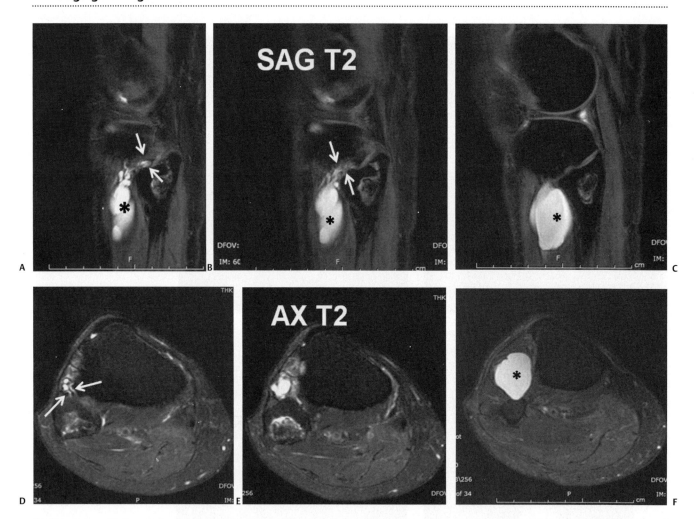

(A–F) A circumscribed, cystic, hyperintense T2 focus (*asterisk*) extends from the tibiofibular articulation (*between arrows*) and tracks into the peroneal musculature. A bone infarct is incidentally noted in the fibular head.

■ Differential Diagnosis

- **Peroneal nerve sheath ganglion:** A cystic lesion that is contiguous with the proximal tibiofibular articulation and is embedded within the peroneus muscles combined with the clinical presentation points to this diagnosis.
- *Synovial cyst*: This is not a common location or path of extension for a synovial cyst adjacent to the knee.
- *Myxoid neoplasia*: These lesions do not have a growth pattern that extends from the proximal tibiofibular joint. They typically appear more complex on T2 weighted images and can display internal enhancement.

■ Essential Facts

- Juxta-articular ganglia are quite common. Around the knee, ganglia may be located in any of the extra-articular soft tissues and commonly are associated with the medial and lateral origins of the gastrocnemius muscle. When

arising from the tibiofibular articulation, a ganglion usually represents dissection of fluid into an articular branch of the peroneal nerve. Less frequently, ganglia in this region may be related to vascular adventitial cysts from the capsular artery. Patients with mass lesions in this region may present with pain or symptoms of nerve entrapment. The lesion compresses the peroneal nerve and its branches, resulting in footdrop and paresthesias over the dorsum of the foot.

✔ Pearls & ✘ Pitfalls

- ✔ Muscle atrophy, fat infiltration, and increased signal on fluid-sensitive sequences may be present in the peroneal musculature with long-standing cysts.
- ✘ It may not be possible to discern between a ganglion and a vascular cyst by magnetic resonance imaging.

Case 98

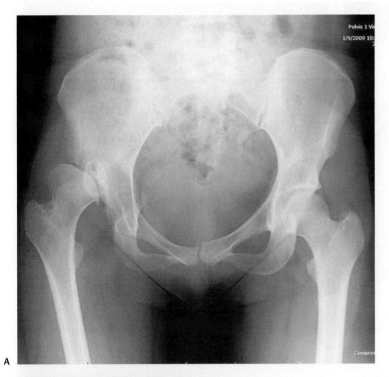

A

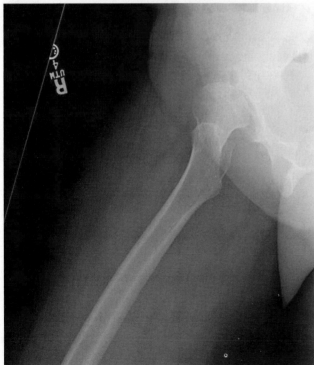

B

■ Clinical Presentation

A 32-year-old woman presents with chronic pain in the right hip.

■ Imaging Findings

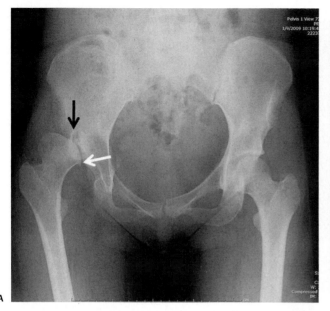 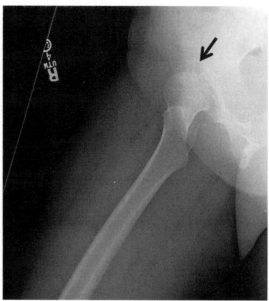

(A,B) Radiographs of the pelvis and right hip show a hypoplastic/dysplastic-appearing lateral acetabular roof containing sclerosis and cystic change (*black arrows*). This process allows superior subluxation of the femoral head, which is shortened and remodeled with an inferior osteophyte (*white arrow*). The left hip is normal.

■ Differential Diagnosis

- **Developmental hip dysplasia:** Unilateral superior subluxation of the hip secondary to an underdeveloped acetabulum is representative of developmental hip dysplasia.

■ Essential Facts

- In developmental hip dysplasia, the acetabulum partially covers the femoral head. In severe cases, superior subluxation of the hip is present.
- The center–edge angle is used to quantify acetabular coverage of the femoral head.
- The angle is formed by two lines, each originating at the center of the femoral head; one line extends vertically, and the second extends to the lateral acetabulum.
- Coverage of the femoral head is considered adequate if the angle measures ≥ 25 degrees. The cause of this condition is controversial.
- It most likely develops in utero and is related to the fetal position. The process is typically unilateral.
- Patients present with anterior inguinal pain, painful clicking, transient locking, and instability of the hip.
- This condition is more common in women and may progress to osteoarthrosis and superior subluxation if untreated.

✔ Pearls & ✘ Pitfalls

- ✔ Developmental hip dysplasia is more common in the left hip and can be associated with labral tears along the anterosuperior quadrant of the acetabulum.
- ✘ Neuromuscular diseases may radiographically mimic this condition.

Case 99

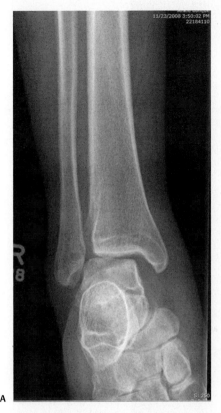

A

■ Clinical Presentation

A 32-year-old man presents with pain in the right ankle that began after a fall the previous night.

Further Work-up

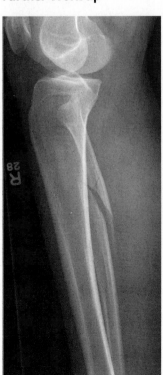

B

■ Imaging Findings

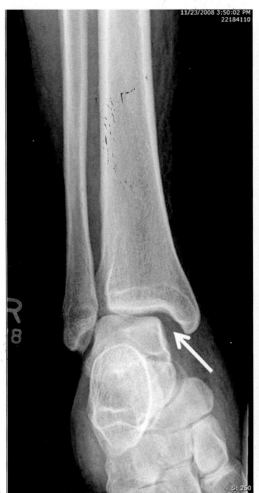 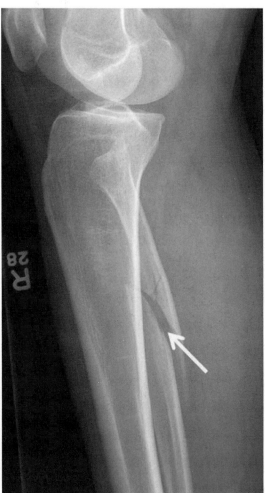

(A) Radiograph of the ankle shows widening of the medial clear space (*arrow*) with surrounding soft-tissue swelling. No fracture is evident. **(B)** A lateral radiograph of the tibia and fibula displays a spiral fracture (*arrow*) through the proximal third of the fibular diaphysis.

■ Differential Diagnosis

• *Maisonneuve fracture:* Widening of the medial clear space and a fracture through the proximal third of the fibular diaphysis are distinct features of this entity.

■ Essential Facts

• A Maisonneuve fracture is an eversion injury of the ankle that presents with medial malleolar tenderness on examination. Widening of the medial clear space secondary to rupture of the deltoid ligament may be the only finding in the ankle. Alternatively, medial and/or posterior malleolar fractures may be seen in the absence of a lateral malleolar fracture. The syndesmosis is typically injured, and a proximal fibular spiral fracture is present. This is considered an unstable injury.

✔ Pearls & ✘ Pitfalls

✔ Suspect this diagnosis in the setting of no visible ankle fracture and widening of the medial clear space of > 5 mm.

✘ Static ankle films may show normal alignment with an isolated nondisplaced medial malleolar fracture.

Case 100

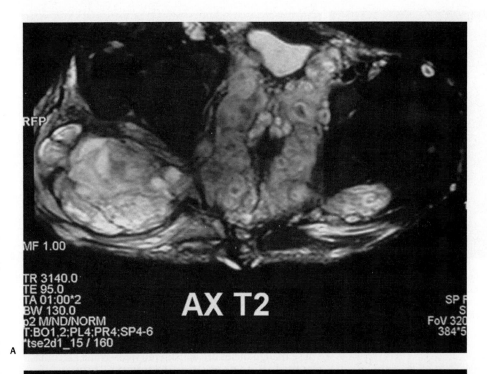

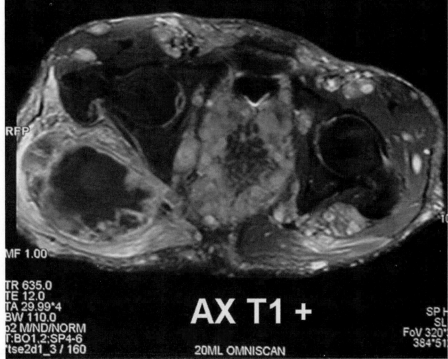

■ Clinical Presentation

The patient is a disfigured 32-year-old man with an enlarging gluteal mass on the right side.

■ Imaging Findings

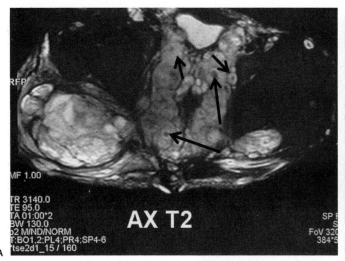

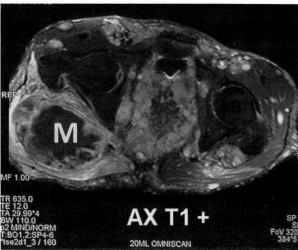

(A,B) Axial magnetic resonance (MR) images of the pelvis reveal multiple rounded masses along the expected course of the lumbosacral plexus with peripheral high T2-weighted MR signal intensity (*short arrows*) and central low T2 signal intensity (*long arrows*)

consistent with the "target sign." A dominant mass (*M*) is seen over the right gluteal region with a central area of necrosis containing high T2 signal intensity without contrast enhancement.

■ Differential Diagnosis

• ***Neurofibromatosis type 1 (NF1) with a malignant peripheral nerve sheath tumor (MPNST):*** This patient's history in combination with the plexiform masses replacing the lumbosacral plexus and displaying a "target sign" on T2-weighted MR imaging is pathognomonic for NF1. The dominant enlarging necrotic mass in the right gluteal region is characteristic of malignant degeneration.

■ Essential Facts

• NF1 is one of the most common genetic diseases. It is inherited as an autosomal-dominant trait and is associated with mutation of a gene on chromosome 17.
• Patients typically present with cutaneous lesions, scoliosis, and mental deficiency.
• The hallmark of NF1 is the plexiform neurofibroma.
• The plexiform neurofibroma represents diffuse intraneural neoplasia in a long nerve segment whose branches show tortuous expansion.
• The gross appearance has been described as a "bag of worms."
• The "target sign" represents peripheral myxomatous fluid with increased T2 signal intensity enclosing central fibrous tissue with low T2 signal intensity.
• A dominant lesion showing rapid growth accompanied by the acute onset of pain, motor weakness, and sensory deficits can indicate transformation to an MPNST.
• The estimated prevalence of malignant transformation is ~5%.

• These malignancies are considered high-grade sarcomas. Eighty percent of patients with MPNSTs and NF1 are male.
• Characteristics of malignant degeneration on MR images include a dominant mass with hemorrhage and/or necrosis.

✔ Pearls & ✗ Pitfalls

✔ Multiple neural lesions demonstrating a "target sign" on T2-weighted imaging with plexiform morphology is pathognomonic for NF 1. MPNSTs most commonly involve major nerve trunks, including the sciatic nerve, brachial plexus, and sacral plexus.
✗ Early dedifferentiation of a neurofibroma to an MPNST may not be evident on imaging.

Further Readings

Case 1

Andrews CL. From the RSNA Refresher Courses. Radiological Society of North America. Evaluation of the marrow space in the adult hip. Radiographics 2000;20(Spec No):S27–S42

Feldman F. Musculoskeletal radiology: then and now. Radiology 2000; 216(2):309–316

Manaster BJ. From the RSNA Refresher Courses. Radiological Society of North America. Adult chronic hip pain: radiographic evaluation. Radiographics 2000;20(Spec No):S3–S25

Case 2

Downey EF Jr, Curtis DJ, Brower AC. Unusual dislocations of the shoulder. AJR Am J Roentgenol 1983;140(6):1207–1210

Case 3

Dinauer PA, Brixey CJ, Moncur JT, Fanburg-Smith JC, Murphey MD. Pathologic and MR imaging features of benign fibrous soft-tissue tumors in adults. Radiographics 2007;27(1):173–187

Case 4

Jacobson JA, Girish G, Jiang Y, Resnick D. Radiographic evaluation of arthritis: inflammatory conditions. Radiology 2008;248(2):378–389

Sommer OJ, Kladosek A, Weiler V, Czembirek H, Boeck M, Stiskal M. Rheumatoid arthritis: a practical guide to state-of-the-art imaging, image interpretation, and clinical implications. Radiographics 2005;25(2):381–398

Case 5

Campbell SE, Sanders TG, Morrison WB. MR imaging of meniscal cysts: incidence, location, and clinical significance. AJR Am J Roentgenol 2001;177(2):409–413

Fox MG. MR imaging of the meniscus: review, current trends, and clinical implications. Radiol Clin North Am 2007;45(6):1033–1053, vii

Case 6

Andrews CL. From the RSNA Refresher Courses. Radiological Society of North America. Evaluation of the marrow space in the adult hip. Radiographics 2000;20(Spec No):S27–S42

Case 7

O'Connor EE, Dixon LB, Peabody T, Stacy GS. MRI of cystic and soft-tissue masses of the shoulder joint. AJR Am J Roentgenol 2004;183(1):39–47

Tirman PF, Feller JF, Janzen DL, Peterfy CG, Bergman AG. Association of glenoid labral cysts with labral tears and glenohumeral instability: radiologic findings and clinical significance. Radiology 1994;190(3):653–658

Case 8

Camacho MA. The double posterior cruciate ligament sign. Radiology 2004;233(2):503–50415516620

Case 9

Resnik CS. Wrist and hand injuries. Semin Musculoskelet Radiol 2000;4(2):193–204

Case 10

Daftary A, Haims AH, Baumgaertner MR. Fractures of the calcaneus: a review with emphasis on CT. Radiographics 2005;25(5):1215–1226

Lee P, Hunter TB, Taljanovic M. Musculoskeletal colloquialisms: how did we come up with these names? Radiographics 2004; 24(4):1009–1027

Case 11

Mann FA, Wilson AJ, Gilula LA. Radiographic evaluation of the wrist: what does the hand surgeon want to know? Radiology 1992;184(1):15–24

Oneson SR, Scales LM, Erickson SJ, Timins ME. MR imaging of the painful wrist. Radiographics 1996;16(5):997–1008

Case 12

Sonin A. Fractures of the elbow and forearm. Semin Musculoskelet Radiol 2000;4(2):171–191

Case 13

Andrews CL. From the RSNA Refresher Courses. Radiological Society of North America. Evaluation of the marrow space in the adult hip. Radiographics 2000;20(Spec No):S27–S42

Zurlo JV. The double-line sign. Radiology 1999;212(2):541–542

Case 14

Diel J, Ortiz O, Losada RA, Price DB, Hayt MW, Katz DS. The sacrum: pathologic spectrum, multimodality imaging, and subspecialty approach. Radiographics 2001;21(1):83–104

Case 15

Deutsch A, Resnick D. Eccentric cortical metastases to the skeleton from bronchogenic carcinoma. Radiology 1980;137(1 Pt 1):49–52

Case 16

Resnik CS. Wrist and hand injuries. Semin Musculoskelet Radiol 2000;4(2):193–204

Sonin A. Fractures of the elbow and forearm. Semin Musculoskelet Radiol 2000;4(2):171–191

Case 17

Robbin MR, Murphey MD. Benign chondroid neoplasms of bone. Semin Musculoskelet Radiol 2000;4(1):45–58

Case 18

Newman JS, Newberg AH. Congenital tarsal coalition: multimodality evaluation with emphasis on CT and MR imaging. Radiographics 2000;20(2):321–332, quiz 526–527, 532

Case 19

Resnik CS. Wrist and hand injuries. Semin Musculoskelet Radiol 2000;4(2):193–204

Sofka CM, Potter HG. Magnetic resonance imaging of the wrist. Semin Musculoskelet Radiol 2001;5(3):217–226

Case 20

Fox MG. MR imaging of the meniscus: review, current trends, and clinical implications. Radiol Clin North Am 2007;45(6):1033–1053, vii

Case 21

Mulligan ME. Ankle and foot trauma. Semin Musculoskelet Radiol 2000;4(2):241–253

Hunter TB, Peltier LF, Lund PJ. Radiologic history exhibit. Musculoskeletal eponyms: who are those guys? Radiographics 2000; 20(3):819–836

Case 22

Levine SM, Lambiase RE, Petchprapa CN. Cortical lesions of the tibia: characteristic appearances at conventional radiography. Radiographics 2003;23(1):157–177

Smith SE, Kransdorf MJ. Primary musculoskeletal tumors of fibrous origin. Semin Musculoskelet Radiol 2000;4(1):73–88

Case 23

Jacobson JA, Girish G, Jiang Y, Resnick D. Radiographic evaluation of arthritis: inflammatory conditions. Radiology 2008;248(2):378–389

Case 24

Resnik CS, Seo GS. Wrist and hand injuries. Semin Musculoskelet Radiol 2000;4(2):193–204

Rosner JL, Zlatkin MB, Clifford P, Ouellette EA, Awh MH. Imaging of athletic wrist and hand injuries. Semin Musculoskelet Radiol 2004;8(1):57–79

Totterman SMS, Seo GS. MRI findings of scapholunate instabilities in coronal images: a short communication. Semin Musculoskelet Radiol 2001;5(3):251–256

Case 25

Beltran J, Kim DH. MR imaging of shoulder instability injuries in the athlete. Magn Reson Imaging Clin N Am 2003;11(2):221–238

Case 26

Rosenberg ZS, Beltran J, Bencardino JT. From the RSNA Refresher Courses. Radiological Society of North America. MR imaging of the ankle and foot. Radiographics 2000;20(Spec No):S153–S179

Case 27

Tirman PFJ, Smith ED, Stoller DW, Fritz RC. Shoulder imaging in athletes. Semin Musculoskelet Radiol 2004;8(1):29–40

Tuite MJ. MR imaging of sports injuries to the rotator cuff. Magn Reson Imaging Clin N Am 2003;11(2):207–219, v

Case 28

Tigges S, Fajman WA. Injuries about the knee and tibial/fibular shafts. Semin Musculoskelet Radiol 2000;4(2):221–239

Case 29

Beltran J, Kim DH. MR imaging of shoulder instability injuries in the athlete. Magn Reson Imaging Clin N Am 2003;11(2):221–238

Ridpath CA, Wilson AJ. Shoulder and humerus trauma. Semin Musculoskelet Radiol 2000;4(2):151–170

Case 30

Bancroft LW, Kransdorf MJ, Menke DM, O'Connor MI, Foster WC. Intramuscular myxoma: characteristic MR imaging features. AJR Am J Roentgenol 2002;178(5):1255–1259

Ly JQ, Bau JL, Beall DP. Forearm intramuscular myxoma. AJR Am J Roentgenol 2003;181(4):960–960

Case 31

Hubbard AM. Imaging of pediatric hip disorders. Radiol Clin North Am 2001;39(4):721–732

Case 32

Hunter TB, Peltier LF, Lund PJ. Radiologic history exhibit. Musculoskeletal eponyms: who are those guys? Radiographics 2000;20(3): 819–836

Case 33

Bancroft LW, Peterson JJ, Kransdorf MJ. Cysts, geodes, and erosions. Radiol Clin North Am 2004;42(1):73–87

Manaster BJ. From the RSNA refresher courses. Total hip arthroplasty: radiographic evaluation. Radiographics 1996;16(3):645–660

Taljanovic MS, Jones MD, Hunter TB, et al. Joint arthroplasties and prostheses. Radiographics 2003;23(5):1295–1314

Case 34

Parman LM, Murphey MD. Alphabet soup: cystic lesions of bone. Semin Musculoskelet Radiol 2000;4(1):89–101

Case 35

Bennett DL, Ohashi K, El-Khoury GY. Spondyloarthropathies: ankylosing spondylitis and psoriatic arthritis. Radiol Clin North Am 2004;42(1):121–134

Jacobson JA, Girish G, Jiang Y, Resnick D. Radiographic evaluation of arthritis: inflammatory conditions. Radiology 2008;248(2):378–389

Case 36

Bansal A. The dripping candle wax sign. Radiology 2008;246(2):638–640

Case 37

Murphey MD, Sartoris DJ, Quale JL, Pathria MN, Martin NL. Musculoskeletal manifestations of chronic renal insufficiency. Radiographics 1993;13(2):357–379

Wittenberg A. The rugger jersey spine sign. Radiology 2004;230(2):491–492

Case 38

Parman LM, Murphey MD. Alphabet soup: cystic lesions of bone. Semin Musculoskelet Radiol 2000;4(1):89–101

Case 39

Murphey MD, Carroll JF, Flemming DJ, Pope TL, Gannon FH, Kransdorf MJ. From the archives of the AFIP: benign musculoskeletal lipomatous lesions. Radiographics 2004;24(5):1433–1466

Case 40

Murphey MD, Robbin MR, McRae GA, Flemming DJ, Temple HT, Kransdorf MJ. The many faces of osteosarcoma. Radiographics 1997;17(5):1205–1231

Case 41

Jacobson JA, Girish G, Jiang Y, Sabb BJ. Radiographic evaluation of arthritis: degenerative joint disease and variations. Radiology 2008;248(3):737–747

Case 42

Patel K, Bhuiya T, Chen S, Kenan S, Kahn L. Epidermal inclusion cyst of phalanx: a case report and review of the literature. Skeletal Radiol 2006;35(11):861–863

Case 43

Resnik CS. Wrist and hand injuries. Semin Musculoskelet Radiol 2000; 4(2):193–204

Case 44

Rosenberg ZS, Beltran J, Bencardino JT. From the RSNA Refresher Courses. Radiological Society of North America. MR imaging of the ankle and foot. Radiographics 2000;20(Spec No):S153–S179 PubMed

Case 45

Feldman F. Musculoskeletal radiology: then and now. Radiology 2000; 216(2):309–31610924543
Manco LG, Schneider R, Pavlov H. Insufficiency fractures of the tibial plateau. AJR Am J Roentgenol 1983;140(6):1211–1215

Case 46

Pao DG. The lateral femoral notch sign. Radiology 2001;219(3):800–801
Sanders TG, Medynski MA, Feller JF, Lawhorn KW. Bone contusion patterns of the knee at MR imaging: footprint of the mechanism of injury. Radiographics 2000;20(Spec No):S135–S151

Case 47

Kransdorf MJ, Smith SE. Lesions of unknown histogenesis: Langerhans cell histiocytosis and Ewing sarcoma. Semin Musculoskelet Radiol 2000;4(1):113–125

Case 48

Flemming DJ, Murphey MD. Enchondroma and chondrosarcoma. Semin Musculoskelet Radiol 2000;4(1):59–71

Case 49

Dinauer PA, Brixey CJ, Moncur JT, Fanburg-Smith JC, Murphey MD. Pathologic and MR imaging features of benign fibrous soft-tissue tumors in adults. Radiographics 2007;27(1):173–187

Case 50

Sanders TG, Medynski MA, Feller JF, Lawhorn KW. Bone contusion patterns of the knee at MR imaging: footprint of the mechanism of injury. Radiographics 2000;20(Spec No):S135–S151

Case 51

Ejindu VC, Hine AL, Mashayekhi M, Shorvon PJ, Misra RR. Musculo-skeletal manifestations of sickle cell disease. Radiographics 2007; 27(4):1005–1021

Case 52

Koyama T, Ueda H, Togashi K, Umeoka S, Kataoka M, Nagai S. Radio-logic manifestations of sarcoidosis in various organs. Radiographics 2004;24(1):87–104

Case 53

Runyan BR, Bancroft LW, Peterson JJ, Kransdorf MJ, Berquist TH, Ortiguera CJ. Cyclops lesions that occur in the absence of prior anterior ligament reconstruction. Radiographics 2007;27(6):e26

Sheldon PJ, Forrester DM, Learch TJ. Imaging of intraarticular masses. Radiographics 2005;25(1):105–119

Case 54

Berquist TH. Osseous and myotendinous injuries about the knee. Radiol Clin North Am 2007;45(6):955–968, vi

Case 55

Llauger J, Palmer J, Rosón N, Bagué S, Camins À, Cremades R. Nonsep-tic monoarthritis: imaging features with clinical and histopatho-logic correlation. Radiographics 2000;20(Spec No):S263–S278

Case 56

Thomas RD, Fairhurst JJ, Clarke NM. Madelung's deformity masquer-ading as a bone tumour. Skeletal Radiol 1993;22(5):329–331

Case 57

Hunter TB, Peltier LF, Lund PJ. Radiologic history exhibit. Mus-culoskeletal eponyms: who are those guys? Radiographics 2000;20(3):819–836
Lee P, Hunter TB, Taljanovic M. Musculoskeletal colloquialisms: how did we come up with these names? Radiographics 2004; 24(4):1009–1027
Stevens MA, El-Khoury GY, Kathol MH, Brandser EA, Chow S. Imaging features of avulsion injuries. Radiographics 1999;19(3):655–672

Case 58

Hunter TB, Peltier LF, Lund PJ. Radiologic history exhibit. Mus-culoskeletal eponyms: who are those guys? Radiographics 2000;20(3):819–836
Lee P, Hunter TB, Taljanovic M. Musculoskeletal colloquialisms: how did we come up with these names? Radiographics 2004; 24(4):1009–1027
Stevens MA, El-Khoury GY, Kathol MH, Brandser EA, Chow S. Imaging features of avulsion injuries. Radiographics 1999;19(3):655–672

Case 59

Ben-Menachem Y, Coldwell DM, Young JW, Burgess AR. Hemor-rhage associated with pelvic fractures: causes, diagnosis, and emergent management. AJR Am J Roentgenol 1991;157(5):1005–1014
Yoon W, Kim JK, Jeong YY, Seo JJ, Park JG, Kang HK. Pelvic arterial hemorrhage in patients with pelvic fractures: detection with contrast-enhanced CT. Radiographics 2004;24(6):1591–1605, discussion 1605–1606

Case 60

Murphey MD, Fairbairn KJ, Parman LM, Baxter KG, Parsa MB, Smith WS. From the archives of the AFIP. Musculoskeletal angioma-tous lesions: radiologic-pathologic correlation. Radiographics 1995;15(4):893–917

Case 61

Beaman FD, Peterson JJ. MR imaging of cysts, ganglia, and bursae about the knee. Radiol Clin North Am 2007;45(6):969–982, vi
Lee P, Hunter TB, Taljanovic M. Musculoskeletal colloquialisms: how did we come up with these names? Radiographics 2004; 24(4):1009–1027

Case 62

Fox MG. MR imaging of the meniscus: review, current trends, and clinical implications. Radiol Clin North Am 2007;45(6):1033–1053, vii

Case 63

Ashman CJ, Klecker RJ, Yu JS. Forefoot pain involving the metatarsal region: differential diagnosis with MR imaging. Radiographics 2001;21(6):1425–1440

Harty MP. Imaging of pediatric foot disorders. Radiol Clin North Am 2001;39(4):733–748

Case 64

Jacobson JA, Girish G, Jiang Y, Sabb BJ. Radiographic evaluation of arthritis: degenerative joint disease and variations. Radiology 2008;248(3):737–747

Case 65

Phillips CD, Pope TL Jr, Jones JE, Keats TE, MacMillan RH III. Nontraumatic avulsion of the lesser trochanter: a pathognomonic sign of metastatic disease? Skeletal Radiol 1988;17(2):106–110

Case 66

Murphey MD, Smith WS, Smith SE, Kransdorf MJ, Temple HT. From the archives of the AFIP. Imaging of musculoskeletal neurogenic tumors: radiologic-pathologic correlation. Radiographics 1999;19(5):1253–1280

Case 67

Karabulut N, Ariyurek M, Erol C, Tacal T, BalkanciF. Imaging of "iliac horns" in nail-patella syndrome. J Comput Assist Tomogr 1996;20(4):530–531

Case 68

Manaster BJ. From the RSNA Refresher Courses. Radiological Society of North America. Adult chronic hip pain: radiographic evaluation. Radiographics 2000;20(Spec No):S3–S25

Petersilge CA. From the RSNA Refresher Courses. Radiological Society of North America. Chronic adult hip pain: MR arthrography of the hip. Radiographics 2000;20:S43–S52

Case 69

Yu KK, Hawkins RA. The prostate: diagnostic evaluation of metastatic disease. Radiol Clin North Am 2000;38(1):139–157, ix

Case 70

Murphey MD, Choi JJ, Kransdorf MJ, Flemming DJ, Gannon FH. Imaging of osteochondroma: variants and complications with radiologic-pathologic correlation. Radiographics 2000;20(5):1407–1434

Case 71

Lee P, Hunter TB, Taljanovic M. Musculoskeletal colloquialisms: how did we come up with these names? Radiographics 2004;24(4):1009–1027

Rao SK, Wasyliw C, Nunez DB Jr. Spectrum of imaging findings in hyperextension injuries of the neck. Radiographics 2005;25(5):1239–1254

Case 72

Llauger J, Palmer J, Rosón N, Bagué S, Camins À, Cremades R. Nonseptic monoarthritis: imaging features with clinical and histopathologic correlation. Radiographics 2000;20(Spec No):S263–S278

Monu JUV, Pope TL Jr. Gout: a clinical and radiologic review. Radiol Clin North Am 2004;42(1):169–184

Case 73

Deliganis AV, Baxter AB, Hanson JA, et al. Radiologic spectrum of craniocervical distraction injuries. Radiographics 2000;20(Spec No):S237–S250

Munday TL, Johnson MH, Hayes CW, Thompson EO, Smoker WR. Musculoskeletal causes of spinal axis compromise: beyond the usual suspects. Radiographics 1994;14(6):1225–1245

Case 74

Jacobson JA, Girish G, Jiang Y, Resnick D. Radiographic evaluation of arthritis: inflammatory conditions. Radiology 2008;248(2):378–389

Sommer OJ, Kladosek A, Weiler V, Czembirek H, Boeck M, Stiskal M. Rheumatoid arthritis: a practical guide to state-of-the-art imaging, image interpretation, and clinical implications. Radiographics 2005;25(2):381–398

Case 75

Andrews CL. From the RSNA Refresher Courses. Radiological Society of North America. Evaluation of the marrow space in the adult hip. Radiographics 2000;20(Spec No):S27–S42

Manaster BJ. From the RSNA Refresher Courses. Radiological Society of North America. Adult chronic hip pain: radiographic evaluation. Radiographics 2000;20(Spec No):S3–S25

Case 76

Cothran RL Jr, Helms C. Quadrilateral space syndrome: incidence of imaging findings in a population referred for MRI of the shoulder. AJR Am J Roentgenol 2005;184(3):989–992

Helms CA. The impact of MR imaging in sports medicine. Radiology 2002;224(3):631–635

Robinson P, White LM, Lax M, Salonen D, Bell RS. Quadrilateral space syndrome caused by glenoid labral cyst. AJR Am J Roentgenol 2000;175(4):1103–1105

Case 78

Boles CA, el-Khoury GY. Slipped capital femoral epiphysis. Radiographics 1997;17(4):809–823

Case 79

Restrepo CS, Lemos DF, Gordillo H, et al. Imaging findings in musculoskeletal complications of AIDS. Radiographics 2004;24(4):1029–1049

Case 80

Kransdorf MJ, Stull MA, Gilkey FW, Moser RP Jr. Osteoid osteoma. Radiographics 1991;11(4):671–696

Case 81

Jacobson JA. Musculoskeletal sonography and MR imaging. A role for both imaging methods. Radiol Clin North Am 1999;37(4):713–735

Oneson SR, Scales LM, Erickson SJ, Timins ME. MR imaging of the painful wrist. Radiographics 1996;16(5):997–1008

Case 82

Anderson MW. MR imaging of the meniscus. Radiol Clin North Am 2002;40(5):1081–1094

Fox MG. MR imaging of the meniscus: review, current trends, and clinical implications. Radiol Clin North Am 2007;45(6):1033–1053, vii

Case 83

Beaman FD, Peterson JJ. MR imaging of cysts, ganglia, and bursae about the knee. Radiol Clin North Am 2007;45(6):969–982, vi

Jacobson JA. Musculoskeletal sonography and MR imaging. A role for both imaging methods. Radiol Clin North Am 1999;37(4):713–735

Case 84

Kaewlai R, Avery LL, Asrani AV, Novelline RA. Multidetector CT of blunt thoracic trauma. Radiographics 2008;28(6):1555–1570

Miller LA. Chest wall, lung, and pleural space trauma. Radiol Clin North Am 2006;44(2):213–224, viii

Case 85

Bancroft LW, Peterson JJ, Kransdorf MJ, Nomikos GC, Murphey MD. Soft tissue tumors of the lower extremities. Radiol Clin North Am 2002;40(5):991–1011

Murphey MD, Gross TM, Rosenthal HG. From the archives of the AFIP. Musculoskeletal malignant fibrous histiocytoma: radiologic-pathologic correlation. Radiographics 1994;14(4):807–826, quiz 827–828

Case 86

Beaman FD, Kransdorf MJ, Menke DM. Schwannoma: radiologic-pathologic correlation. Radiographics 2004;24(5):1477–1481

Murphey MD, Smith WS, Smith SE, Kransdorf MJ, Temple HT. From the archives of the AFIP. Imaging of musculoskeletal neurogenic tumors: radiologic-pathologic correlation. Radiographics 1999;19(5):1253–1280

Case 87

Metz VM, Schimmerl SM, Gilula LA, Viegas SF, Saffar P. Wide scapholunate joint space in lunotriquetral coalition: a normal variant? Radiology 1993;188(2):557–559

Case 88

Miller SL, Hoffer FA. Malignant and benign bone tumors. Radiol Clin North Am 2001;39(4):673–699

Smith SE, Kransdorf MJ. Primary musculoskeletal tumors of fibrous origin. Semin Musculoskelet Radiol 2000;4(1):73–88

Case 89

Beall DP, Googe JD, Moss JT, et al. Magnetic resonance imaging of the collateral ligaments and the anatomic quadrants of the knee. Radiol Clin North Am 2007;45(6):983–1002, vi

Case 90

Connolly SA, Connolly LP, Jaramillo D. Imaging of sports injuries in children and adolescents. Radiol Clin North Am 2001;39(4):773–790

Case 91

Sookur PA, Naraghi AM, Bleakney RR, Jalan R, Chan O, White LM. Accessory muscles: anatomy, symptoms, and radiologic evaluation. Radiographics 2008;28(2):481–499

Wright LB, Matchett WJ, Cruz CP, et al. Popliteal artery disease: diagnosis and treatment. Radiographics 2004;24(2):467–479

Case 92

Gupta KB, Duryea J, Weissman BN. Radiographic evaluation of osteoarthritis. Radiol Clin North Am 2004;42(1):11–41, v

Jacobson JA, Girish G, Jiang Y, Sabb BJ. Radiographic evaluation of arthritis: degenerative joint disease and variations. Radiology 2008;248(3):737–747

Case 93

Naimark A, Miller K, Segal D, Kossoff J. Nonunion. Skeletal Radiol 1981;6(1):21–25

Case 94

Gielen JL, Blom RM, Vanhoenacker FM, De Schepper AMA, Van de Vijver K. An elderly man with a slowly growing painless mass in the soft tissues of the lower leg: case presentation. Skeletal Radiol 2008;37(4):335, 337–338

HolobinkoJN, Damron TA, Scerpella PR, Hojnowski L. Calcific myonecrosis: keys to early recognition. Skeletal Radiol 2003;32(1):35–40

Case 95

Andrews CL. From the RSNA Refresher Courses. Radiological Society of North America. Evaluation of the marrow space in the adult hip. Radiographics 2000;20(Spec No):S27–S42

Steinbach LS. "MRI in the detection of malignant infiltration of bone marrow"—a commentary. AJR Am J Roentgenol 2007;188(6):1443–1445

Case 96

Diel J, Ortiz O, Losada RA, Price DB, Hayt MW, Katz DS. The sacrum: pathologic spectrum, multimodality imaging, and subspecialty approach. Radiographics 2001;21(1):83–104

Case 97

Beaman FD, Peterson JJ. MR imaging of cysts, ganglia, and bursae about the knee. Radiol Clin North Am 2007;45(6):969–982, vi

Spinner RJ, Scheithauer BW, Desy NM, Rock MG, Holdt FC, Amrami KK. Coexisting secondary intraneural and vascular adventitial ganglion cysts of joint origin: a causal rather than a coincidental relationship supporting an articular theory. Skeletal Radiol 2006;35(10):734–744

Case 98

Manaster BJ. From the RSNA Refresher Courses. Radiological Society of North America. Adult chronic hip pain: radiographic evaluation. Radiographics 2000;20(Spec No):S3–S25

Petersilge CA. From the RSNA Refresher Courses. Radiological Society of North America. Chronic adult hip pain: MR arthrography of the hip. Radiographics 2000;20(Spec No):S43–S52

Case 99

Hanson JA, Fotoohi M, Wilson AJ. Maisonneuve fracture of the fibula: implications for imaging ankle injury. AJR Am J Roentgenol 1999;173(3):702

Case 100

Murphey MD, Smith WS, Smith SE, Kransdorf MJ, Temple HT. From the archives of the AFIP. Imaging of musculoskeletal neurogenic tumors: radiologic-pathologic correlation. Radiographics 1999;19(5):1253–1280

Index

Note: Locators refer to case number. Locators in **boldface** indicate primary diagnosis.